Sis, You Got This!

Sis, You Got This!

From Surviving to Thriving as a Minority Speech-Language Pathologist

With Foreword by Vicki Deal-Williams, MA, CCC-SLP

Barbara Fernandes, MS, CCC-SLP

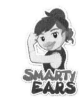

Smarty Ears LLC
Dallas, TX

Sis, You Got This! From Surviving to Thriving as a Minority Speech-Language Pathologist

Cover Design by Abanoub Sobhy
Illustration by Violetta Itskova
Editors: April Alvis, Arielle Hadfield, and Terilyn Julkes
Printed in the United States

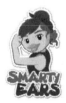

www.smartyearsapps.com

Digital ISBN: 979-8-88525-326-0
Paperback ISBN: 978-0-578-26191-1
Hardcover ISBN: 978-0-578-26192-8

Table of Contents

Acknowledgments

Even though this book was written in twenty-eight days, it was the culmination of thirty-eight years of life supported by individuals who believed in and supported me so that I could one day share these stories with you. This is the section of the book designed to honor them.

First, I want to honor my family. My children, Victor and Alice, who fill my heart every day with hope for a more accepting world with their kindness and genuine embrace for equity and justice. They now can know just a bit more about their mommy. My husband and best friend, Jonathan Fernandes, who always held the fort when I needed to get things done, was always ready to read over my work, and was always willing to take the kids to a park to support me in making this book a reality. I know I could not have done this without your support. I love you, Handsome.

I also want to honor my father, Alcides Fernandes, an ordinary, humble man with wisdom beyond several lifetimes. He made me believe in dreams. He is the type of human I can only aspire to be every single day.

To the women who looked back, saw me, and threw a rope of hope my way, Desirée Begrow, Rosangela Boyd, Vicki Deal-Williams, Melanie Johnson, Catherine Crowley, Irmgard Payne, Pat Brandt, Veronica De La Cruz, Doanne Ward-Williams; and the women from my Minority Student Leadership Program (MSLP) support system, who have always cheered me on, saved a seat at their table for me, mentioned my name for opportunities, answered my calls for help, or looked me in the eye and said, "Don't let this dim your light." I remember you, and I honor your role too. This is also to the many other SLPs who have contributed to my career by trusting in me and supporting my work over the years. Especially the Smarty Ears authors who have trusted and joined me in my efforts to make speech therapy resources more dynamic.

My deepest gratitude to the contributors of this book, the sixteen other minority speech-language pathologist women who shared their hearts, stories, and tears with me: Maria Claudia Franca, DM (anonymous contribution), Ebony Green, Enjoli Richardson, Jamila Perry Harley, Leila Regio, Mai Ling Chan, Michelle Hernandez, Michelle Posner, Pelesia Fields, Ramya Kumar, Tamala Close, Pang Tao Moua, Phuong Lien Palafox, Yarimar Díaz Rodríguez, and Yao Du. Your experiences touched and pushed me to think beyond my own experiences. Thank you, ladies, for trusting me to handle your words with care, even when we knew so little about what this book was turning into.

I also want to acknowledge a trio of women whose actions sparked the fire in me to make this book a reality: Yarimar Díaz Rodríguez, Vicki Deal-Williams, and Dr. Kia Johnson. You had no idea of the impact of your actions and courage. This book is a result of the impact the three of you had on me. Your actions completed an important healing cycle for me. Thank you!

Finally, I want to acknowledge that I am the fruit of many different programs designed to give me a chance in life, despite my background. I would not have gone to college in Brazil without a federally funded public university. I would not have made it to the US without an initiative by the Brazilian and American Education Departments to sponsor me, and I would not have stayed in this field without the Minority Student Leadership Program. These programs have allowed me to thrive and reach my full potential. I honor and acknowledge them today and forever.

Foreword

A month or so after the announcement that I would become the next CEO of the American Speech-Language-Hearing Association (ASHA), I found myself in the lobby of the Marriott Marquis in Washington, DC in the midst of the 2021 ASHA Convention, surrounded by a throng of well-wishers offering congratulations for taking on this new role. I've been filled with a level of gratitude and emotions that defy words (which is saying a lot for a seasoned speech-language pathologist). In looking back on my path to this point, it would be inauthentic to withhold that there have been moments of loneliness, self-doubt, bouts of imposter syndrome, as well as comments from some questioning my qualifications for the role. At those times, I've been blessed to be able to call on a small group of sister-friends who provide an effortless form of therapy and offer edifying and encouraging words that push aside that doubt and those questions, and replace it with *Sis, You Got This!*

Every audiologist or speech-language pathologist I know who is a person of color can easily recount experiences of being made to feel invisible, less than, or like an outsider at some point(s) along their professional journey. We can each tell stories that should have never been lived experiences, and current BIPOC students in Communication Sciences and Disorders (CSD) are reporting similar incidents and encounters. Unfortunately, the reality is that with 218,000 members, ASHA is a microcosm of our larger society. Way too many individuals routinely express their biases and –isms resulting in hurt and offense that has had dire consequences for our professions.

Having worked to effect change over the years on diversity and inclusion within our discipline, it pains me deeply that we have to live with the myth of the 8%, but it's become ASHA folklore. ASHA's non-White racial composition does add up to about 8.5%, but there is an additional 6% of the ASHA constituency comprised of individuals who identify as Hispanic/Latina/o/x. Because there is overlap in those two groups, we cannot add those numbers together. ASHA's racial/ethnic diversity makeup is actually somewhere between 8.5% and 14.5%. So, while we have increased our racial/ethnic composition, it is nowhere near the increase we need and want.

So why would I still highly recommend this discipline to someone aspiring to become an audiologist or SLP? Because there are individuals like Barbara Fernandes among us who make us better! Barbara uses *Sis, You Got This!* to bring to life the importance of the support we can provide to each other that helps each of us persevere, rise above, and contribute to the discipline of human communication and related disorders in ways that would otherwise not be possible. She helps us realize that the real story is not in our protracted progress or the trials themselves. The real story is in the triumphs, the thriving, and the victory over seemingly insurmountable odds.

Barbara offers a level of transparency and vulnerability that comes to life on the pages that follow. She bares her soul and what would be soul-crushing defeats to the average person. She recounts her life, leadership experiences, and her growth through multiple encounters when she felt she couldn't persevere, including one when our paths first crossed back in 2005, to a full circle moment in 2021, when she was the one offering a hand up to a CSD student at the end of her SLP rope. You'll see through the stories she and her contributors share that others are placed in your path for a reason and that there is power in our struggles. This book offers the inspiration that so many need so they know they are not alone and that there are others who have trod this path successfully. And, while we're working to re-pave that path, you too can navigate it and flourish. Fernandes offers insight into those things about you that make you perfect for our professions, because of your background, and proves that you can shine in our field. The strength and courage you see in these women's experiences and responses will empower you to press on and create your own reality instead of allowing others to define your future.

As I take the helm at ASHA, I find myself reflecting now not on our trials, but instead on our potential and collective capability. We need you and your contributions to help design a future and to evolve into the best discipline we can possibly be. This book is the reminder that we all need to be here for each other to hush the whispers inside and outside of our heads that can deter us from achieving our true destiny.

Vicki R. Deal-Williams, MA, CCC-SLP, FASAE, CAE

Barbara Fernandes

Preface

Who Is This Book for, and Why Do You Need It?

"Some of us make it out. But the game is played with loaded dice.
I wish I had known more, and I wished I had known it sooner."
Ta-Nehisi Coates

When I tell you about this Latina speech-language pathologist immigrant, you might be led to think that she has always had it together in order to achieve all that she has. She arrived in the US at twenty-one and didn't speak much English. Now, she speaks multiple languages, owns two successful businesses, and has developed sixty apps and an entire diverse communication symbol set. She has even been a guest speaker at several conventions around the world. You might ask yourself, "How can I relate to someone like this? I'm barely treading water. People like her must have all their ducks in a row. They have always had a plan. They are the type of people who have known their professional career path since they were in kindergarten and have developed a detailed fifteen-year plan for everything. Right?"

Let me tell you, she didn't, and she was playing with loaded dice. This book tells my story. I am that Latina immigrant. I didn't always know what I was doing, and I changed my mind many times about which direction I wanted to go; but most importantly, I had no awareness of just how loaded my dice were until a few years ago. My journey was filled with adversity, a weak set of cards, and a background that was often perceived as less than, but I am thriving. Now that I am here, I'm looking back and extending my hand (well, more like extending the reach of my words) to say:

Sis, you can do it too.

I wrote this book for you. Yes, you. I want you to thrive and reach the top of your mountain as well. You who don't quite feel like you belong. You who may feel, at times, that you can't keep going anymore. You who feel the weight of your background and all that it comes with. You who dream of becoming a speech-language pathologist but do not know if you have it in you to keep fighting the fights that should have been won a long time ago. You who feel like progress may come but it will be too late for you because you need that progress right here and right now.

You are me, and I am you. This book is also for you who have earned your degree—your undergraduate, your master's, or your PhD—but are still trying to find your voice in this field; or you may have found your voice but are still afraid to use it. This book is also for you who, despite your latest degree or your highest position, and despite your few or many successes, still feel like you have not found the joy that comes with discovering your worth in this profession. It is for you who may still have a lot of healing to do from traumatic experiences as you worked your butt off to become who you are. And it is for you who are still dealing with not being recognized for the level of your accomplishments because you do not look like those who are in a position to give it. This book is also for you who are trying to start your own business and do your own thing in the speech and language field, but have quickly learned that having worked so hard to earn your degree won't prevent you from being disappointed by how much harder it is to make it as a minority woman in this field.

Lastly, this book is for you who, despite all your accomplishments, still can't control the tears from falling when the very people who made you feel small over a decade ago appear out of nowhere at a convention and still manage to make you feel less than them, smaller than them, or less wise than them.

I am also writing this book for that version of myself who timidly attended a presentation by Vicki D. Williams (ASHA's Chief Staff Officer for Multicultural Affairs) and Catherine Crowley at the American Speech and Hearing Association (ASHA) Convention in 2005 about the treatment that international students were facing in communication sciences and disorders (CSD) programs across the United States. That version of me sat in the back, sobbing as she related to the presenters' examples of discrimination against accented speech in CSD programs. That twenty-two-year-old Barbara needed this book. That version of me had no idea of her worth. She had no idea of the many gifts she already had in her that would one day revolutionize this field, partly thanks to her unique past experiences. She needed the words in this book sixteen years ago to help her keep going. Today, I need these words to continue to heal.

This is not a book filled with research references, pie charts, and data that you may find hard to connect with. This book is filled with stories of my experiences and the things I learned from them. It is filled with confessions about my journey, my mistakes, and the effects of others on me. I am confident that you will find that you and I have a lot in common. In that, I want you to feel the power of the connections of our shared experiences. I want you to feel the power of knowing that no matter how lonely you may feel as a minority SLP, there is a group of women who see you, and we are doing all we can to make your dice a little less loaded. In order to do that, I recruited other minority SLP women to share a bit of their hearts, experiences, lessons, and perspectives with you as well. You will learn their stories and their lessons throughout this book too. These women are my safe space, and as you read our hearts, you will feel that you are not so different from us. Just like you, each of us brings unique perspectives, and I strongly believe that's the exact reason why we thrive. We struggled. We cried. We broke down. This book is my way of telling you to keep going and to show you the power of representation, which is far from cliché. I believe that you have a lot to contribute to this field, and the world, just as you are.

This book is for you who are looking for a sense of belonging in one of the whitest professions in the United States (with a staggering 91.5% of SLPs being white, only behind veterinarians, farmers, and mining machine operators [According to the US Bureau of Labor]). This book is my attempt to give you a sense that you are not alone. You have the power to make your very own contributions in our field through your unique experiences and background.

I am now on the verge of turning forty years old, and I have accomplished enough for several lifetimes. Despite my many accomplishments and contributions, I am still dealing with microaggressions, sexism, and systemic exclusions that you would think I wouldn't have to deal with anymore. Let me tell you, bullshit will find a way to affect us until we die, so we can't count on it not happening. While I am a lot better at it than I used to be, I am still learning how to process and respond every time it happens. It has helped me to become aware of the dice and the games that people played to attempt to keep me from playing. I wish I had this awareness sooner. I don't want you to wait as long as I did to find your self-worth. You are worthy as you are, but if you learn to harness your experiences and your strengths, you will become unstoppable.

If you and that young 2005 model of me were sitting next to each other at the ASHA presentation, I am sure that we could have had a chat and I would have told you, "I can't wait until I finish earning this degree and show them all that I can do." To which you might have replied, "Me too!"

Girl, you don't have to wait. In fact, I insist that you don't. You got this!

Heck! Earning that graduate degree did not show them, and apparently, I didn't even show myself all the power I had. That goalpost kept moving, and I did it to myself. I kept waiting for someone to validate my worth. I defined my self-worth by how much I had endured, achieved, and contributed. Your self-worth should not be put on hold while you are enduring trauma for pursuing a degree in communication disorders. I want you to see your worth right now; not when you earn your next degree, or move to your new job, get promoted or start your new business. Earning your degree is stressful as shit, but your background as a minority student or professional should not add to that stress.

Now that you know that this book was written for you, I want to tell you why you need it. You may need this book because you have heard from your boss or your clinical supervisor that the way you look or talk is triggering fears in your clients because they associate that accent or skin color with "bad people," and you didn't even know how to respond. You just felt like giving up. I want to show you the many ways you can recognize how deeply those hurtful words hit your soul, then silence that painful voice you keep repeating in your head, find your strengths, and take action to shine and to thrive.

You need this book because you may not yet have realized that you have allies who may not look or talk like you but have experiences similar to yours and can empathize with you. Empathy (as opposed to sympathy) is powerful. This is where you may find your chosen family within the profession, which is what happened for me. Finding that group of people who will mention your name in a room full of opportunities, who will stand by you when you have a breakdown during an ASHA Convention, or who will say, "That's my girl" when you are succeeding is as important as your degree. We are out here, waiting to do that for you.

You need this book because I don't want you to give up. I want you to keep going. I want you to thrive! In order to do that, I believe that you need to do as much internal work as the professional work that you do. This includes having more awareness of the toxic people around you or environments you find yourself in, being aware of how they affect you, breaking away from cycles of trauma responses, and finally, unlocking and playing to your strengths.

It is easy to imagine we would be doing better as a profession. After all, we belong to a field in which the fundamental classes teach about language proficiency, second language learning, language and culture, bilingualism, and many other things that seem like they should help the majority of our peers and colleagues do better. Unfortunately, this is not always the case. *Knowing* better does not necessarily mean *doing* better. We all have implicit bias, and it is a bitch. Many people lack the awareness of their own internal bias. This prevents them from making necessary changes.

Topics of racial bias and cultural sensitivity toward our clients have been, for some time, a very prominent subject in our field. Yet, the discussion on these biases and their impact on CSD students and colleagues of color, immigrants, and other minorities has been largely absent. While you might have hoped that the skills learned and discussed for one population would be generalized to include another, they are not. Some people may not know what to do or how to act toward people of differing backgrounds. Nonetheless, I believe in giving most people some level of grace. I am willing to give them perspective to support necessary change. I hope you will have the courage to join me in helping the majority group of SLPs do better too.

Finally, you need this book because people are often surprised when I tell them that I never had an ultimate plan for building what I managed to accomplish in life. I love telling them that I wasn't even sure about the small steps I was taking, but I took them anyway; now, I am living my best life. I want you to hear from minority SLPs who are thriving like me and see yourself in us. Read our struggles, our pain, our doubts, and know that you don't have to have things figured out to thrive. You already have what it takes to thrive too. You will also read the stories of other SLPs who are still struggling. May you find awareness of your own struggle through their words, and may our collective stories become the lighthouse you will remember in times of darkness.

But before we keep going, I want to acknowledge that I am not an anthropologist, sociologist, or an expert in the topic of race or ethnicity. I am merely someone who is experiencing life as a Latina immigrant who became an SLP in the United States. The stories in this book reflect that journey, my perception of specific events, and the lessons I took from it. With that said, I understand that some industries have moved away from the use of the word "minorities," and some individuals even consider it offensive and prefer using other terms such as, "minoritized," "marginalized," and others. Trust me: I hear you, and I dwelled on it for a long time. I have decided to stay with the term "minority" because it has always had a connotation of oppression and discrimination, regardless of whether or not the group in question was represented in larger numbers. I chose it especially because, in our field, the term "minority" applies to both the numerical and "minoritized." As you will soon see, one particular group in our field may be the minority in number, but they are not minoritized, and we need to move away from numerical discussions soon enough.

Before you move forward, look back at the cover and tell yourself, "I am not an ugly duckling. I am a swan!" You are a swan in the field where you were made to feel inferior because you are different. I invite you to continue this journey with me as I retell the times I went from animal to animal, listening to, "You don't belong here, go away," until I finally discovered that I am a swan.

Enjoy.

Part One: **Surviving**

Chapter 1:

Let's Get Acquainted

"Because true belonging only happens when we present our authentic, imperfect selves to the world, our sense of belonging can never be greater than our level of self-acceptance." Brené Brown

I have had days when I was trying to get out of a certain mood or looking for advice, so I Googled "how to have a difficult conversation" or "how to fit in." I promise that typing those words and many other "how to" searches didn't sound as stupid then as it sounds now. The end result was often the same: a cheap, easy-to-read article filled with bullet points on how to achieve something. It often had no information on who wrote it or their credibility to be giving that advice. Worse, these articles were often written without much context to actually help me remember the one good piece of advice among everything else. With this book, I wanted to offer more. I want you to connect with these words as you read about my failures, thought processes, and moments I almost gave up. I want you to actually remember the stories before you read my takeaways. I hope you also form your own takeaways. Stories are memorable; cheap bullet points are easy to forget. I want you to remember, so I am telling you a lot of stories.

By the end of this book, you will have gotten to know me quite a bit. You may even feel like you and I have become BFFs. When you know someone's deepest hurt and pain and their process out of it, you end up getting a glimpse of their soul. As you read and get to know me, while reflecting on how you and I may share similar experiences, I want you to feel that you have a new ally. As you navigate these chapters, I want to give you so much of me that when we meet in person, we will already have a connection, and you will have someone with whom you can share your difficult experiences. This is Introduction to Barbara 101. It is meant to give you enough information about me that you can trust we will have each other's backs. It is intended to give you detailed insight on why I decided to write this book, and it is intended to help you change your life by the time you're done reading it.

Oi, Amiga! That's how you say, "Hi, Friend," in Portuguese. I was born in Salvador, the third largest city in Brazil. Salvador is a coastal city with beautiful beaches. It has the largest concentration of African descendants in the world, outside of Africa. Because of its African influence, Salvador has a very unique culture. Think of it as the New Orleans of Brazil. I lived in Salvador until I was twenty-one years old. Brazil is a large country, and like in the US, people born in different areas have different regional cultures. The same is true of Brazilian immigrants in the US.

My birth mother gave me up for adoption as a fourteen-day-old baby. Abandonment and adoption have played a big role in my life and my behaviors, and they required healing. For most of my life, the answers to medical predispositions were filled with unknowns. When it came to heritage, there was another huge gap in my knowledge bank. Because of this, I knew early a thing or two about looking around and feeling like you don't quite belong. Thanks to living in the time of affordable genetic heritage discovery, I learned a lot about my ancestry background. In 2012, I did my first genetic test with AncestryDNA, and my composition was 55% European, 40% Sub-Saharan African, and 5% Indigenous. In 2017, I did 23andMe, and my results came in as 68% European (mostly Portuguese and Spanish), 23% Sub-Saharan African (mostly Congolese), and 8% East Asian and Indigenous. Just like most Brazilians in the northeast, I am a mix of the Brazilian Indigenous communities and those who arrived in Brazil in the 1500s.

The couple that adopted me had three biological sons of their own—the youngest being twelve years old when I arrived. My adoptive father was a truck driver, and my adoptive mother ran a small tourist gift shop. I went to a private school, had a roof over my head, food, and a loving father. I grew up in a neighborhood that was also very diverse in terms of race, socioeconomic status (to a degree), and educational level. However, to American standards, my neighborhood would probably be considered a neighborhood of poverty. I had neighborhood friends who were a part of a family of twelve siblings without a father figure all living in a two bedroom rental, but I also had neighbors whose parents were doctors and lawyers. I was somewhat in the middle of that scale; my house had one TV and two bathrooms, the family car was at least from the 60s, and not a single room in my house had AC.

In my neighborhood, there was a strong sense of community. If I was hungry, I could easily ring the doorbell of my neighbor and have dinner there. If you have lived in any country in Latin America, you may possibly relate to this intense sense of community—the kind where it feels like everyone is constantly up in your business, but also ready to help as if you were their family. It makes for an incredibly positive sense of belonging and a complete lack of privacy at the same time.

My childhood was far from unremarkable. Like many of you, I am still healing from the trauma—for example, the abandonment by my biological mother. I reconnected with her this year and learned that she was in a state of modern-day slavery. She was locked in as a stay-at-home maid for a wealthy white family without any compensation or permission to make contact with her family. These challenging circumstances forced her to hand me over. My heart ached, for her and me, as I learned about the unthinkable stories she shared with me. Traumatic experiences will push us to feel and react to things a certain way our entire lives or until we are ready to face them and heal.

I won't bore you with details about Brazil; you are better off buying plane tickets and visiting. Among other things, Brazil is a source of pride for me because both federal and state funded colleges are free without compromising quality. This is one of the reasons I am sitting in my comfortable living room in a different country. College accessibility allowed me, and those who could never afford a private university, to access higher education and claim our space under the sun.

The free college debate in the United States has been quite heated in the current political scenario; people have the impression that it is a free

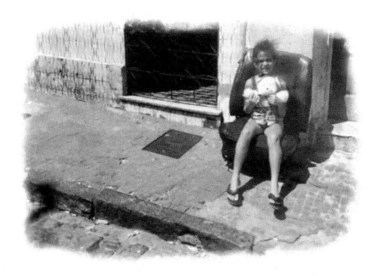

That's me sitting across from my home.

handout to unqualified students. In reality, the public colleges in Brazil are the hardest colleges to be accepted into. They made it possible for me to contribute to society in ways I could never have imagined, but more on that later. I am not interested in convincing you that debt-free college accessibility is important for social mobility, but I would like to share more about my experience with it.

As you can imagine, high quality, fully funded colleges are highly competitive; even the rich kids would rather spend money buying a car for college than paying for college tuition. In fact, the public universities in Brazil are the highest ranking educational institutions in the country. In order to get admitted to any program for any college in Brazil, you are required to take a multi-day exam and rank amongst the top. When I finished high school and applied in 2001, there were only twenty spots for the speech-language pathology and audiology program and 4,000 applicants. That makes roughly one spot for every 200 applicants. These numbers highlight the fact that in Brazil, higher education is not accessible for all. While the numbers have significantly improved since private colleges became more prevalent, they still do not measure up to the US by any stretch of the imagination.

I was seventeen years old when I was accepted into one of the speech-language and audiology programs at the Universidade Federal da Bahia (Federal University of Bahia). The program was academically challenging but extremely rewarding. It was a brand-new program at my university; my class was the third speech pathology class in my state. All of my professors were from out of state. They were figuring things out on the fly, and that had its own set of challenges. For example, many of my first semester foundational classes, such as Sociology Applied to Speech Pathology, Psychology Applied to Speech Pathology, Intro to Audiology, Genetics, Biophysics, and Dentistry applied to Speech Pathology, were taught by non SLPs.

During the four year program, I was set to graduate with a degree in both speech pathology and audiology. It was an intensive program; students had classes from sunrise to sunset most days. Some days, I was in class until 8 p.m. That was the price I had to pay to earn two degrees in four years. Things got more intense the second year when I began my externship and began working on my thesis, which I would be required to defend and present to a panel in order to receive my degree.

During my undergraduate program, I also engaged in leadership roles by becoming president of the student council for two years. As the program was in its inception, it was extremely important to have engaged students making sure things could progress. We had a dentist as the chair of the speech department because there were no post-graduate SLPs available for the position. Yes! A dentist. I know.

Participating in leadership roles as a student allowed me to start developing skills that I continue to use today. If you are a student, consider doing the same at your university. In order to thrive, you will have to develop some leadership skills, and what better time to get your feet wet than during your undergraduate or graduate program?

During my final year in college, my father was diagnosed with cancer, and that shook my world immensely. My father, who was already older, was forced to stop working. His truck sat in front of our home day and night. Financially, it meant that in order to get to college every day, I had to walk one hour there and back. It meant that I had to eat breakfast at home, and many days, I would not eat again until I was back home. Walking the streets at night in a developing country with a high crime rate was a major safety concern. They say these things are resilience builders; I am not sure how I feel about that.

One day, without knowing that my entire life was about to change, I stumbled upon a flyer that was recruiting students from speech pathology and special education programs to take part in an exchange program. It would include a semester at Temple University in Philadelphia called "**Promoting the Inclusion of Persons with Disabilities in Society Through Assistive Technology: Culturally Appropriate Solutions.**" The program planned to bring four American students to Brazil to learn how Brazil implemented alternative communication, which at the time was primarily without any technology. Meanwhile, four Brazilian students would travel to the US to learn about the AAC technology used and bring that knowledge back. This exchange student program was sponsored by the Brazilian Department of Education in conjunction with the American Department of Education.

As you can imagine, the selection process to participate in a program in the US with all expenses paid was highly competitive. During our first meeting, the program coordinators revealed a set of qualifying tests and rating scales. The scales included English skills, which I had just recently started studying. Most of my peers were from upper middle class families. They drove to classes in their cars, and many had already visited the US before as tourists. That meant that many of them had been studying English their entire lives. This was not my case.

I was clearly the least qualified person when it came to English skills in comparison to my peers seeking that same opportunity. At that point, I could have decided to give up against the competition, and looking back, I can't believe I didn't. I chose to take massive action and decided to score the highest on the other items on their selection scale. It is my hope that you will also choose not to give up when you feel at a disadvantage against people who were dealt better cards than yours.

Before I tell you where that story goes, I want to address the elephant in the chapter: you might be wondering how someone who barely had money to take a bus to class was learning English. The answer comes with one of the very first pieces of advice I will give you: **take as many opportunities that appear!**

Remember how I said that I was at college all day long with barely any time to breathe? Yes! That's a thing. Among the many classes I took, one of them was Biophysics. My professor, Luis Claudio, needed teaching assistants for his class. In free public universities, professors don't have the funds to pay teaching assistants. Luckily for me, Professor Claudio was creative in finding students to assist him. He owned an English school and offered his teaching assistants a free semester. "Sign me up," I said! At the time, I had no idea what I would do with whatever English I would learn. I had no intention of going to the US, nor could I imagine a day that I would actually use that new skill, but I was not going to let that opportunity pass by. So I became a Biophysics teaching assistant in my second year of college in exchange for one semester of English school.

Once that semester at the English school was over, I would have to pay if I wanted to continue to attend. I obviously could not afford to pay that tuition, so I needed a different solution. At the time, my professor did not have a website for his school, so I proposed that I create one for him.

I don't remember how or why I taught myself to design websites, but I knew enough to trade that skill for another semester learning English. **Knowledge is power. It will become an incredible currency when you don't have currency in the bank.**

I began building the website in 2002. You may be too young to know this, but at that time, people were charged by the minute to use the internet. Each night, I waited until after midnight—when the internet was free—in order to build the website that covered my tuition to learn English.

Another difference back then was that there were no drag and drop tools to build a website. It was a complex process with coding and formatting. But that's what it took for me to learn English, and thereby earn a spot in the English school; so I signed up, and I handled it. I hope you learn as soon as yesterday that you can learn anything you set your mind to and that knowledge will become your currency, just like it became mine.

The only reason I even had a chance and was ready to amplify other areas of my life when that selection process came up was because I pushed myself to use my knowledge to trade for more knowledge. The English course was a great opportunity for me; however, it was only two hours per week. You and

I both know how difficult it is to learn any language when you are only doing it for two hours a week.

When the exchange student selection committee revealed the results, I was ecstatic to find that I was one of the four students selected. You might be wondering how I overcompensated for my very limited to non-existent English skills. Let me let you in on another secret: I don't remember exactly what items were considered besides English level and our GPA. I know there were other parameters; however, I was mainly aware of my desperate need to overcompensate for my developing English skills. Despite my god-awful memory, I clearly remember the faces of the speech pathology students who reached the final selection stage with me. As I mentioned earlier, unlike me, all of them were from the upper class and had been to the US on vacation before. That fact didn't scare me; it pushed me even harder to show what I could do despite my circumstances.

That initiative helped me land my second big shot into a path to thrive in life.

When I heard that English proficiency levels were qualifying prerequisites, I did not just say, "never mind." My best friend at the time, Adriana, who I was hoping would join me on this journey to have fun adventures in a new country—who probably also had much better English skills than me— gave up and became self conscious about her limited English proficiency. I, on the other hand, doubled down on my books and audio CDs. I studied ahead for hours on end every single night. If you know a thing or two about learning languages, you know there's no telling how much progress I actually made here. However, I was learning vocabulary skills specifically related to TOFEL. I would stay up until midnight so that I could use my dial-up internet to do the free practice online tests. But the important thing to note, here, is the state of mind to push through and give your all when something matters.

Initiative. That is one of my favorite words in the English dictionary. If I had to place a percentage value on what actually weighed the most, I have no doubt that my initiative was the biggest reason I was selected. During the very first meetings, I constantly offered to create effective ways for the coordinators to communicate with the candidates. I created a Listserv group, so they could easily communicate meetings and details and many other things that made their lives easier. I developed creative solutions for many of the issues they presented. I became their go-to tech girl. Since this was a technology grant, I am inclined to imagine they must have been very impressed with my tech solutions. I made their lives easier, and I had the initiative.

Once I learned that I was one of the four students selected for this opportunity, I will confess that I was not sure I was going to take it. I actually hesitated. My father was sick, my family was struggling to make ends meet, and I was so close to finally graduating, becoming the first person in my family to graduate from college, and having financial freedom. I could have graduated in six months if I didn't take on that opportunity to participate in the exchange student program. If I decided to accept the opportunity, that would mean that upon returning, I would have to wait at least another six months—but likely a whole year—to be able to join another graduating class offering the coursework that I needed in order to graduate.

It was difficult to make sense of the emotions in my head. When you are twenty-one years old and six months away from graduating and leaving it all behind, there is a mix of fear for the unknown and excitement for the possibilities. No matter how much you hear this on American television, not everyone has a dream to actually live in the USA. I have always dreamed of traveling the world, but the thought of spending six months away from everything I'd known had never occurred to me before. I considered backing out many times.

But eventually, I got on a plane, as a twenty-one-year-old girl with a suitcase full of dreams, to live for the next six months in a brand-new country, wondering what that experience would add to my professional life. I had no idea that it was not just adding to my professional life, but it was adding even more to who I am.

Reflection Question: How do the first twenty-one years of your life shape how you react to difficult experiences in your CSD program or as a clinician?

Barbara Fernandes

Chapter 2:

The Immigrant SLP

"Do you know what a foreign accent is? It's a sign of bravery."
Amy Chua

When you come to study in the US from another country, you are considered an international student. This is what I became when I landed in Washington DC in August of 2004. Besides paying a much more expensive tuition, international students face significant challenges that are unique to being in the communication sciences and disorders field. This chapter is dedicated to sharing my unique experiences as an international student from Latin America.

If you are not an international student, don't skip forward. The stories in this chapter will serve you in a few ways. First, you will discover a whole group of individuals, like me, whom you may identify with on a completely different level. My stories of discrimination, bias, and skepticism regarding my abilities are something that you and I may share, even if you didn't immigrate to the United States, and even if English is your first language. Second, learning about the struggles of immigrants, you may realize that you hold some biases that are worth looking into. Third, we need you as an ally, and you need us. In a field that is composed of so few minorities, unity is the only way forward. Immigrants with an accent have their own fair share of struggles both as immigrants and as English as Second Language

(ESL) learners—or even simply as learners who speak a different dialect of English. I hope that in hearing my story, you will become an ally too.

Let me make this clear: this section of the book *is not* designed for me to give you definitions of a non-native accent or to lay out the research on how much more difficult accented speech is to be understood by individuals with communication disorders. You can easily find great resources on that elsewhere, such as ASHA's technical report by Crowley, Catherine & Levy, Erika & Mahendra, Nidhi & Deal, Vicki. (2011). The Clinical Education of Students With Non-Native Accents - ASHA Professional Issues Statement. 10.7916/d8-bmab-4t40 (Crowley et al., 2011).

This book is meant to be read while listening to your favorite inspirational music artist, which for me is India Arie.

Now that we got that out of the way, let's get back to our heart-to-heart stories. Guys, landing on US soil for the first time is magical. It is like landing directly into a movie. I felt like I had won life right then and there. Bless my heart, I was so unprepared to handle the things that I was about to experience. I was completely unaware of what I looked like, what I sounded like, or how my English was perceived. Despite this, I felt like the most privileged person in the world.

My very first wake-up call was at the airport. Our flight from DC to Philly was canceled, and we were offered a bus from DC to Philly. I quickly realized that all the English I thought I knew was out of the door. Nobody understood what I said, and honestly, I was struggling to understand what everyone else was saying. That was a reality check for me. I thought, "*I am screwed!*"

There were four of us who traveled together for this experience: two were SLP students and two were special education students. All four of us had our own set of goals, plans, and dreams. As we got settled in Philadelphia, we were fortunate enough that both individuals who created the program on the US side were Brazilians. This helped me, as the person needing the most English support, get settled. Dr. Rosangela Boyd, who was a Temple University professor and one of the coordinators of the exchange student program, was the lifeline for the four of us and would later go from being my mentor to becoming my family in the United States. During the semester-long program, I attended a few specific AAC classes, worked as a teaching assistant for some extra income at the Pennsylvania Initiative on Assistive Technology (PIAT), and visited schools for internships specific to AAC. The goal was to become an expert in AAC so that we would be able to bring ideas back to Brazil when the program was over.

For the first four months, my limited English skills prevented me from picking up on the difficult situations I was facing. I had the pleasure to work with incredibly accepting individuals at PIAT, though most of them were not SLPs. They helped move us to our apartment, collected donations for the apartment, and got us settled. Plus, I was on cloud nine! I walked the streets fascinated by the smallest details, such as accessible street crossings, Braille on the campus doors, and even the fact that an adult with cerebral palsy had the means to have a full-time position with speech to text and a wheelchair that seemed out of this world. I felt like I was transported to a world where people with disabilities had accommodations and support to be active members of society. I had never even heard of that before.

I want to share a story, just to give some context as to my level of ignorance about all this back then. Go ahead and laugh out loud now. The very first time I arrived at the public school for my AAC externship, the SLP opened her closet of AAC devices. She had anywhere from twenty to thirty devices in that closet—most of them dead, unused for years, not programmed, or broken. I thought the USA must be so rich to have these amazing devices locked in a closet. If these were the ones not being used, I could not even imagine what devices the kids must be using. Yes, if you didn't laugh out loud before, this is your time.

I share that story because I want to address something that is important for both new immigrant students and those who are not immigrants. We grew up in a different country with different values, different racial dynamics, different educational experiences, and definitely different technology. This story highlights my erroneous bias about how the USA handled AAC. I didn't have the knowledge back then about public school funding nor about how hard AAC devices were to program and all the other inherent contextual information. Coming from Latin America, where my AAC was cutting pictures from magazines because we didn't have a printer, any type of voice output device seemed technologically advanced.

I remember walking around campus at Temple University and being very aware of the racial separations at the cafeteria. There were tables with only Black students, tables with Asian students, and tables with white students. This was also something new for me to experience, and as an outsider who fell from the sky, I had no understanding of the dynamics. In the end, I found myself at a table with other international students, regardless of whatever field we were pursuing. There is a freedom that comes with being able to be yourself and speak English however it comes out when you are around other international students.

If you are a recent immigrant in our field, be aware of the conclusions you are making about your experiences. If you are not an immigrant, know that your immigrant colleague will come with their own set of assumptions, which you will navigate and could assist with.

During the semester as an exchange student, I was making some serious progress with my English skills, thanks to speech-pathology and AAC. I was also picking up a lot more cultural information and expectations of behaviors. One of the coolest coincidences happened in 2004. The ASHA Convention was held in Philadelphia that year, and the four of us were able to attend. How cool is that?

If you have never attended an ASHA Convention, let me tell you that entering a convention center filled with SLPs and audiologists is empowering and unlike anything I ever experienced back home. I am a sensitive person, and I think I got inspired to change the world just by walking through those doors and flipping through the convention planner. Stepping inside the exhibit hall and getting a glimpse of an industry completely designed to develop materials and resources to support individuals with communication disorders is extraordinary. It gave me goosebumps! Even the idea that you would have enough people to have 1,600 presentations all surrounding speech, hearing, and communication disorders is still unbelievably massive to me. I was mesmerized by the numbers and the privilege to walk among that crowd. I felt like the definition of privilege for three days. I thought about my peers back home, my best friend, and how I would never be able to describe the emotions I was feeling and the opportunity I had. I collected the amazing giveaways they passed out, not having a clue that I would soon enough be passing out my own materials in that same hall.

As the semester came to an end, and it was almost time to pack up my bags and go back home, my university in Brazil went on a strike. As a federally funded university, professors went on strike to protest the need to have their salaries increased. That new reality meant that if I returned home, I would have to wait a whole year to resume classes. Those strikes have been known to last months. There was no telling when I would actually be able to graduate if I returned home. This is the part of my story where other women stepped up to help me rise. Dr. Boyd offered to host me if I wanted to transfer my credits to Temple University to complete my undergraduate program in the US. She also offered to pay for the tuition of the remaining semesters. There are moments in life when people look back and reach out to help you; that's what she was doing for me. That's the power each one of us has once we get to where we want to be: to look back and see who is coming behind us, so we can lend our hand and help them get to where they want to be too.

There were a lot of hiccups in the journey from a temporary exchange student to becoming a full-time student aiming for an undergraduate degree. One of the biggest ones was the fact that I had entered the US on a J-1 visa. J-1 is also called an Exchange Visitor visa. Here is what Wikipedia says about these visas:

> "*A J-1 visa is a non-immigrant visa issued by the United States to research scholars, professors and exchange visitors participating in programs that promote cultural exchange, especially to obtain medical or business training within the U.S. All applicants must meet eligibility criteria, English language requirements, and be sponsored either by a university, private sector or government program.*"

Under that visa requirement, I was obligated to return home and spend two years there before ever returning to the US. As I had been sponsored by a governmental program, the requirement was in place because they were investing in people, and they wanted those trained new professionals to return and pay them back with their knowledge. That makes a lot of sense, right? In order for me to stay in the US and finish my undergraduate degree, I had to return home, apply for a new visa, and ask for forgiveness on that requirement, which is exactly what I did. Upon my return to Brazil, I applied for an F-1 Visa, a student visa, explained my story, and I was granted permission to promptly return to the US. I spent my Christmas home, broke off my engagement with my fiancé, and returned to Philadelphia. This time, I was a lot less naive about the roadblocks I might experience ahead, but still full of hope for the future.

Once I arrived back at Temple University, my main goal was to get as many credits as possible transferred from my university in Brazil to Temple in order to reduce the number of remaining credit hours and the cost for me to obtain my undergraduate degree. I was expecting to impress the faculty at Temple when they saw how comprehensive the syllabus I had with me from my university in Brazil was. In order to do that, I translated my transcript and every syllabus for every class, and I asked for personal meetings with each instructor in order for them to inspect the syllabus and decide if my previous coursework was comparable to what they would be teaching in their class. Let me tell you, each one of these meetings was incredibly different from the others, but they had one thing in common: their ability to even entertain waving the coursework requirement was directly related to their past experiences or previous knowledge with other international students or colleagues.

Can you picture yourself going to another country and after six months of learning the language, asking for meetings with a group of the most intimidating people—SLP faculty—to convince them to give you credit for their class without actually attending it? As I look back, I can't imagine the kind of courage it took me to do this. Honestly, I can't believe I did it. But I did. Unfortunately, I wasn't successful each time.

Remember when I said that my coursework in Brazil was extremely comprehensive and focused on speech, language, and audiology? I remember sitting with the Voice Disorders instructor, and it was lovely when he recalled a well-known Brazilian SLP who specialized in voice, Dr. Mara Behlau. He knew that Brazil had an excellent educational level for SLPs, and he signed off on those credit hours. On the other hand, I remember the instructor for Introduction to Audiology, who didn't even care to look at the syllabus, said, "I would never sign off on this, no matter how many credits you have in Audiology." I can still remember her attempt to say how audiology could be different in Brazil. No, ma'am, this is not phonetics. Audiograms are the same anywhere in the world. I had seven audiology classes, plus a lot of actual internship experience, but nonetheless, I still had to take her Introduction to Audiology class. This is a clear example of how important it is for us to check our biases before reaching conclusions. Could she have attempted to do some research before making a decision? Yeah, she could have, but she made up her mind without even putting her eyes on my syllabus. I even offered to take her final exam and have that be the determiner, but she was impenetrable.

The process of earning credits toward my undergraduate degree gave me many more stories to share, but I wanted to share two: one defining moment that pushed me to the brink of changing majors and one story that filled me with shame for years.

During my Language and Culture elective class, the incredibly supportive professor, who was also a minority, though not an SLP, invited the chair of the CSD department for a guest lecture. She started her lecture with a definition of a communication disorder:

"A communication disorder is anything that draws attention to it."

The professor asked in response,

"A foreign accent draws attention to it; is it a communication disorder?"

The chair of the CSD programs replied, "Yes." As the only person with a foreign accent in the room, I could feel every eye turn toward me. I felt naked. I felt shame. I had nowhere to hide. In no time at all, I went from the person who was seeking a degree to help individuals with communication disorders to the one with a disorder. *Is this worth it?* I wondered. *Is this degree worth this humiliation?* I could feel myself losing my self-worth with each passing day. How did I go from being one of the most well-spoken students in a CSD program in Brazil to becoming someone who most faculty would rather be elsewhere?

I had many international student friends in other fields at Temple University; some were getting their PhD or master's degree. They were from all over the world, and they seemed so happy. Why was I struggling so much? Looking back, I know the answer. You know the answer. Back in 2005, only 2.5% of speech and language pathologists were Latinx. At the time, I was completely unaware how that could impact me in any way; I don't even know if I could grasp why that statistic mattered. I don't want you to be as naive as I was. The numbers are better now, but 2016 reminded me that xenophobia is alive and well eleven years later.

I was surviving, and some days felt like I was barely making it. Not because of the academics, which were fairly easy for me, but because of how much of myself would need to disappear in order for me to become the SLP that the Temple faculty wanted to see in me. It was not about feeling different, which was one of the emotional things about life in the USA with so many people from so many places. In fact, that is truly the most beautiful thing in America; you don't see this where I come from. It is, instead, about discovering that you are different in a bad way. It has been sixteen years since, and I still feel emotional as I write this.

No matter how much my English syntax improved, I still sounded like a recent immigrant. I started to view that aspect of myself as a bad thing, and I needed to do whatever it took to make my speech "good." If you have learned anything about me thus far, you know that when I make up my mind, I will push through it. I purchased two to three accent reduction CDs. I would fall asleep every night listening to them in hopes of blending in and sounding just like everyone else. Knowing what I know now about my worth, but still feeling that insecure version of myself, I wanna go back there and hug myself. I started to loathe how I sounded, and in the process, I started to wish to turn into someone I was not. I started to become speechless. I started to believe that I could never accomplish anything in this field if I continued to sound the way I sounded.

"I was at a voice conference in 2019, and during one of the sessions I attended, a team from Brazil was presenting. I heard someone sitting next to me say, "I don't want to listen to that accent," and they left. I was so frustrated. In fact, I heard many comments throughout the convention of people complaining about foreign accents. All of that rubbed me off so much. As someone whose accent occasionally appears when I am more comfortable, I feel like this is an area in our field that I can't possibly belong to." Leila Regio

Like Leila, I attended a voice convention in the summer of 2005 in Philadelphia. I felt exactly like that one person with an accent who noticed people reacting to other accents. I felt looked down on. At this point, I felt ready to be "happy" like my other international student friends, in a different field that was not so focused on changing a part of me that I felt I didn't have much control of. I was ready to switch majors when Dr. Boyd, the program coordinator—and now my host mom—insisted that I attend my second ASHA Convention in San Diego in 2005.

When I actually made it to my second convention in 2005, I was in a completely different state of mind from when I attended the ASHA Convention the previous year in Philadelphia. They were just one year apart, but I was defeated; I felt broken. I was much more aware of the difference between me and everyone else walking around the convention center. Even as I walked around, timidly hiding my speech, I had a feeling that I was hiding this secret that everyone could see. This is a feeling you may still have today as you attend ASHA Conventions. Despite the increase in the percentage of minorities, the numbers are still very low. We still stick out, you know? Among ASHA members and affiliates, less than 14% of us come from racial or ethnic minorities, while only a little over 4.5% of us identify as Hispanic.

I can still feel all the feels of walking around and trying to imagine a world in which someone who sounded like me could ever become an SLP. That was a dream that I thought could never be real. Remember the story of me sobbing during a presentation at the ASHA Convention in the opening remarks of this book? This is the part of my journey where that happened. Looking through the list of presentations, one called my attention: Standards for International Students in CSD Programs. As I sat in the back and listened to the stories those two presenters shared, every word they spoke hit me as if they were talking directly to me. I was emotional, but I tried as much as possible to keep my composure. I couldn't. The emotion was stronger than I. When that session was over, I approached the presenters to chat and thank them for the presentation. At that point, the emotions that I kept bottled up took over me; I could hardly speak because I was crying so hard. I felt so embarrassed talking to them and being unable to hold back my emotions. I shared my experiences, and it felt good to be heard and understood by two SLPs for the very first time. There was power in knowing someone saw me and others like me and was taking steps to make things better for us. However, you know when you are struggling with something in the present and feel like you can't wait for things to get better anymore? You can't wait for people to improve their attitude and see value in you behind your accent, and you just don't want to wait? While I was grateful for what they were doing, it still felt like too little too late for me, but they gave me a little bit of hope.

By the spring of the following year, I earned my undergraduate degree with *Summa Cum Laude* and a GPA of 3.95 (as an ESL student, that

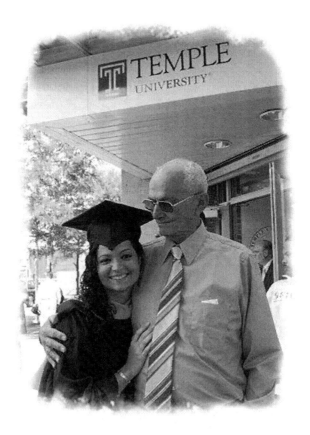

phonetics class kicked my butt). I had made the Dean's List with the second highest GPA in the college of public health. I brought my father from Brazil to witness my graduation. It was his first time leaving the country. He was very frail, and it was the last time I saw him before he passed less than one year later. My father, a truck driver whose highest education was first grade, witnessed one of his kids graduate in the United States. That was pretty awesome. I am saving the tie he used that day to give it to my son one day.

It may not surprise you that despite reaching this milestone, my self-esteem was severely damaged. I arrived in the US as this kickass communicator who was selected for an exchange student program with all expenses paid to represent my country in what felt like a movie. I went from that to becoming someone who "has a communication disorder," and through a series of microaggressions and skepticism, was made to feel inferior to everyone around me. I knew that if I was going to stay in this field, I had to give another university a try. I decided to apply to a program with a bilingual emphasis because I had hopes of finding SLPs who were more accepting of bicultural students elsewhere.

I applied and was accepted to the bilingual master's program at Texas Christian University (TCU) in Fort Worth, Texas with a full scholarship. I was accepted, not because I was a bilingual Portuguese/English speaker, but because I had actually learned Spanish while learning English and working toward my undergraduate degree; I had become a trilingual speaker.

Back home, I had people bragging about how I was living, studying, and graduating in a developed country and how I learned two new languages and was on my way to another degree. In my mind, I had very little faith I could pull this off. Doesn't this say so much about how experiences that degrade who we are impact our perceptions of ourselves? I continued to listen to the accent reduction CDs and practiced daily. However, I applied for a program that I didn't know yet but would significantly alter that state of mind: ASHA's **Minority Student Leadership Program** (MSLP).

Reflection question for faculty: Have you considered your own bias or limited knowledge about other country's academic experiences and how that will shape your interaction with students from that country?

Chapter 3:

Finding Your Support:
Minority Student Leadership Program

"First they came for the socialists, and I did not speak out—
because I was not a socialist.
Then they came for the trade unionists, and I did not speak out—
because I was not a trade unionist.
Then they came for the Jews, and I did not speak out—
because I was not a Jew.
Then they came for me—and there was no one left to speak for me."
Martin Niemöller

In the fall of 2006, I had just returned from a summer public health program in Costa Rica to start my master's program at TCU. A couple of weeks into the program, I received a notification that I had been accepted for the 2006 ASHA's **Minority Student Leadership Program** (MSLP) that I had applied to before moving to Texas. By the time it was time to attend ASHA in November, I was struggling to find my place in this new life, but things had gotten a lot better. I was still working hard to survive, but every new experience and every new win, like being accepted into the master's and MSLP programs, was slowly improving my confidence that maybe I could keep going. I had no idea what to expect from the MSLP program; all I knew was that the program was paying the expenses for me to travel and attend the 2006 ASHA Convention in Miami.

I remember arriving at the hotel in Miami and being paired with my roommate. She was loud, happy, confident, and outspoken. Looking back, unlike me, she scored very high on her extroverted scale.

Another more recent MSLP alum, Leila Regio, shared her roommate experience with me:

> "I was so nervous coming into this roommate situation. We had never met each other, and we are from different backgrounds. However, the moment we met, we instantly connected. Both of us got denied previously, and we tried again. Just hearing what she had already done for racial equity in her college was amazing. It opened my eyes to what so many people were already doing prior to coming into this."
> Leila Regio

During the opening evening reception, I approached someone who I didn't realize I already knew. She was standing by a pillar. I approached her and said, "You look very familiar; I think I already know you from somewhere." She replied that she thought I looked familiar also, but she could not place me either. After a couple of minutes, we both had an aha moment that I will never forget. She was the presenter from the previous year's ASHA Convention presentation in which I sobbed at the back and approached the presenters at the end. That was me and her again. It was a very emotional moment for me, and I dare say for her too. I already looked a little less broken and felt a bit more confident because I was impacted by her a year ago. I didn't know yet, but the MSLP program was her baby.

During the four days of the program at the ASHA Convention, I met and made lifelong friendships with several other minority SLP students. I had no idea there were so many other SLPs with accents in the US. I didn't know there were so many other students who felt like I did. The group was diverse. I even met another Brazilian student, Maria Claudia Franca. I was on cloud nine, feeling like I could be myself among SLPs for the first time in a long time. I had no idea that one day, many of them would become my family in this field. We met people that we could look up to and other people who looked like us and had reached positions many of us would never dream of aiming for. We shared our experiences with each other, and we bonded through those experiences and empathy for each other's struggles. I also remember meeting a Latina professor from a university in California, and when she opened her mouth, it was like music to my ears. Her non-native accent was the icing on the cake that I needed to believe that I could be her one day. The impact that representation can have on society to propel an unknown number of humans to aim for the stars is not cliche. That's what I was experiencing!

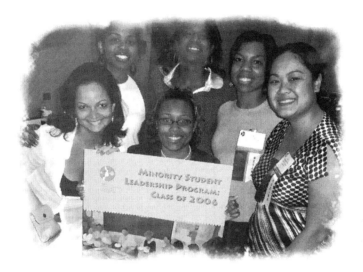

If you are a minority student, please visit the website for the American Speech and Hearing Association and apply. If there is one action item you take away from this reading, I want it to be to apply to the MSLP program. In fact, I want you to close this book right now, close this window on your Kindle or iBooks, open your browser, and check when the next deadline is for the MSLP. Trust me, you will thank me later.

"I attended the MSLP program in 2006, and that was a HUGE support for me in a time when I desperately needed it. They continued to be a support for me for years. They knew so many resources, and they helped me. They told me where to find it. I didn't even know

what NBASLH was. I learned about it during the MSLP program."
DM (Anonymous Contribution)

By the end of the program, I felt empowered, and I felt like I could conquer the world. Those four days were the beginning of the internal work that would carry me to the days that I would write a book to talk about it. Most of it is about doing the internal work that we, as a group who are often met with skepticism, need to do in order to start seeing our true worth. There was so much healing in sharing and listening. I was ready to return to TCU, face the skeptics, face my own ghosts, and become the SLP I was meant to be.

The MSLP program was a two-way street for me, both for my own healing and awareness of my own biases. There is an incredible need for us as individuals to take a good look at our biases toward other minority groups, hence my quote at the beginning of this chapter. Being part of a minority group does not automatically exempt you from bias and prejudice toward other minority groups. There was so much that I didn't know I shared with so many other individuals who looked different from me and had a different story from mine.

We all have preconceived ideas about our own minority group and others. I even have a preconceived bias about Brazilians who come from different parts of the country. There is power in the exercise of acknowledging these biases. As we allow these conversations to happen without judgment, we connect; life is not so lonely anymore. The MSLP program made me feel like I belonged through our shared experiences and the lack of support in our respective programs. It made me feel that I was a little less alone, and my empathy level had grown tenfold. This was not the end to my journey of learning, conquering my biases, conquering my fears, and healing; it was just the beginning.

I am aware, and you should be too, that everyone experiences life differently and because of that, everyone will have their own bias toward other minority groups. While my experience in the MSLP program allowed me to feel like part of a larger group, that apparently was not the experience of everyone. You will see this from the story I am about to tell you, which happened twelve years later, in 2018. I was not planning on attending the

ASHA Convention that year but changed my mind last minute. Hotels were hard to come by, so I ended up rooming with an MSLP alum. I will forever be embarrassed for my lack of response to her comments towards the Black people working at the hotel and her Black students in the city where she worked as an SLP. I roomed with her for one night before finding other friends who would take me in. Just like me, she is part of a minority group, and she participated in the MSLP program; however, she had not yet done the soul search bias work I am asking you to do throughout this book.

The next morning, my friend Ramya Kumar, another immigrant SLP, found me behind a large sign at the convention center in Boston, crying. I was frustrated. I was ashamed of my lack of response. I was angry and felt like I had just let my friends down. Regardless of how much soul searching I had done, I was not prepared to deal with that unexpected behavior from a colleague. I wondered at that moment: if other racially profiled colleagues were openly expressing such horrible sentiments, how badly were the others who have never felt the weight of discrimination?

Regardless of that one setback, my MSLP family has grown as I've gotten to meet other alumni of the program. With each passing year, I have collaborated and cheered them on, and I know that they are doing the same for me. As I was doing my own outreach for this book, I came across this message from 2011 from a fellow MSLP alum and good friend:

> "I have interacted with loads of parents here in NY, and every CE course I take I am constantly recommending your Apps! You are doing an amazing job! I am like your unpaid/unsolicited spokesperson lol. After all, I have to be true to supporting fellow MSLPers. Keep up the great work! Whenever there is a presentation on technology, they usually mention Smarty Ears, and I am always clapping when they do. People came up and asked why I reacted that way, and I gave the whole speech about MSLP and how great you are yadda yadda lol."
> Timberly Leite, MSLP 2006

Over the years, the women I met through this program have been my biggest supporters. I have called them to ask for motherhood advice as well as clinical trial nightmare advice. We have published apps together, applied and received grants, presented in conferences, and they have been the women whose calls for help I will always answer as well. These women have gone places. They are now faculty, chairs of departments, members of ASHA's board of directors, past ASHA Convention co-chairs, National Advisor for NSSLHA, and even chair of the National Black Association for Speech-Language and Hearing (NBASLH).

In 2019, I wanted to honor them and had a special custom illustration made for them to honor our friendship. I cried and made them cry with a whole speech about belonging. These women are the reason I found belonging among minorities, and that's the power of MSLP.

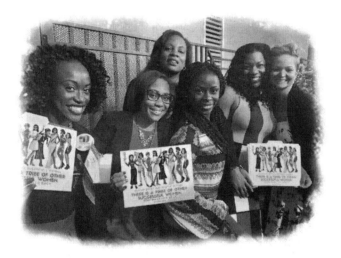

In fact, when I read my friend and colleague Ramya Kumar's contribution to this book, I became even more aware of the importance of this program in making me feel like I have a place to belong in this field:

> "I haven't really connected with groups like the minority SLPs at ASHA or the multicultural caucuses. I feel like a fish out of water there. There is a caucus for Indians, but I don't feel like I belong because I'm on an island of being a DBCD (Dubai Born Confused Desi. Desi is the word in Hindi for Indians, or fellow countrymen. ABCDs are American Born Confused Desis, and FOBs are Fresh off the Boat). There are so many groups amongst Indians alone, that I chose to stay away from that and find my own through other connections." Ramya Kumar

I can absolutely relate to Ramya's feelings from having attended the Hispanic Caucus once in the past and never returning. It made me feel even more grateful for my MLSP sisters for making me feel like I have a place to belong every year I attend the MC2 gatherings at the ASHA Convention. These gatherings always feel like home to me. I believe belonging is a feeling you get when the majority of the place or community welcomes you as you are.

Barbara Fernandes

Chapter 4:

I Am Not Alone

"It's up to all of us—Black, white, everyone—no matter how well-meaning we think we might be, to do the honest, uncomfortable work of rooting it out." Michelle Obama

As much as I am proud of my 25% to 40% Sub-Saharan African genetic makeup (my results varied by each company), I am completely unqualified to bring you the perspective of being a Black SLP in America. The same goes for my 8% East Asian or Indigenous makeup. That's why I reached out to my community and asked them to share a piece of their story with you and me about their own experiences while in school. As I reached out to my colleagues, I offered them two ways to contribute. They could either write their thoughts or schedule some time to chat and be vulnerable with me as I listened to what they had to share and asked questions. As I started this process, I was not prepared for the level of vulnerability, pain, and heartache my friends and colleagues would share with me. I watched some of them cry as they retold their stories. I cried with them. These are not comfortable conversations, but we all need to have more of them. At times, I could see their brains spinning as they were asked to dig deep about things they might not have ever stopped to think about and process on their own. I honor them and their experiences, and I ask you to do the same.

Listening to my close friends and the new friends whose stories you will read here, you will see that we share a surprising number of stories. As an immigrant, learning that people born in the USA, with American English as first language accents, were hearing the same kinds of comments from their CSD professors as I did was hard to fathom. This is why I want you to read the story of Tamala H. Close, a Texas native, who is now the owner of her own private practice. She was one of three African American students in the Southern University A & M's Speech-Language Pathology program, and through the words she shared with me, I can see that we share a lot of very similar experiences.

> "The feelings of isolation were heightened with an experience with one particular professor who made it her duty to identify and diagnose my dialectal difference as a disorder. Being a statistical and cultural outlier wore on my confidence in becoming an exemplary SLP in the field of speech and language pathology. I was constantly questioned regarding how I would effectively treat clients with speech and language disorders if I too was disordered." Tamala H. Close

I know it is 2021, and we have had much more exposure to the struggles of minorities as members of society in this country, but aside from what I heard from my MSLP peeps in 2006, we are not calling each other to hear of SLP-specific situations. Just like I have done for over a decade, these women often brushed off these experiences. I wanted to shed light on them.

During my call with DM, who was a classroom teacher for seven years before becoming an SLP, I asked how her experiences as a Black SLP were different from her experiences as a Black teacher, and here is what she told me:

> "There were definitely fewer Black people in speech than in education, both in the program as well as in the workplace. I am now the only Black woman in my department. There are several Latinas that I feel a strong connection with. In education, I didn't feel the stress of the world against me. The battles I was fighting were for my children. I didn't experience microaggressions in education; the microaggressions were directed toward the children and their families. However, as an SLP, I can feel that I am constantly fighting the fights for myself as a Black SLP." DM

DM shared a story with me from when she attended Mercy College to pursue her master's degree.

"The director of the program was very supportive. She was an Irish immigrant, and she was there for me; it was a safe place. However, I had this one professor who was the head of clinicals and in charge of giving clinical assignments. One semester, I was put on academic probation because I got a C in Neurology class. She called me in her office, and she talked to me as if she was gloating. It felt as if she were happy that I was on probation and said, 'You and your friend are both on academic probation.' I was surprised that she was sharing another student's academic issues with me, but I knew that my friend had also gotten a C in Neurology. Here is the clincher: the person she was calling 'my friend' was the other Black girl in the program that I didn't even get along with. My actual friend was white! She also put me in a placement that I told her would not be a good fit. She replied that I didn't get to choose my placement. She assumed I was friends with the other Black girl, when in fact the white girl who was my friend told me that she was offered the same placement, refused, and was given another placement. The situation turned even more tragic when the interview turned sour and she made me go back and be interviewed yet again. Those scars are things that weigh you down, and I felt helpless as she pushed me around." DM (Anonymous Contributor)

DM's feeling of being targeted as a Black student was not the only story I heard. Pelesia, a Kenyan immigrant, shared a similar story during her time at Lehman College of City University of New York .

"When I got admitted to the CSD program, I was stoked because I was one of the fifteen students accepted into the program out of two hundred students. However, getting admitted was the beginning of a living hell. One particular professor made me constantly feel as if she was out to get me. On one of the papers that I was most proud of, she gave me a B, saying that I had poor grammar, poor punctuation, and picked apart my reference page because it missed a comma. One time, I asked to see the paper of another girl to see what I was doing so differently that was not up to par with what she expected; and my jaw was on the floor. The grammar on that paper was, in my opinion, equivalent to a ninth grader, but to the professor, it was a quality paper. I ended up asking several people to read my papers, including the people at the writing center. I lost confidence that I could write. I would show up at the writing center and they would ask, 'What exactly do you want from us? Because your writing is good.' Eventually, she recommended that I take a writing class. I ended up taking a non-credit with other students who were working toward their GED. I was a graduate student, and I am sitting in a class with GED students. This all from her beating me down and saying that my writing was not of quality.

Eventually, she ended up recommending that I meet with the chair of the program, who is another white woman. I remember sitting with her in the office and she says:

'Pelesia, you might wanna consider a different career path based on what a faculty has informed me about you.'"

Pelesia is not alone in having her writing skills placed under the magnifying glass:

"There was the clinical supervisor who held my report containing blood-red edits. As she handed it back to me, she concisely stated that I wrote poorly because I am an English language learner." Phuong Lien Palafox

"I have always hated that when my writing was poor, everyone always associated it with the fact that I was an English language learner. What if I just wasn't good at writing, just like many people whose English is their first language and their writing is very poor. Why can't I just be treated like them? What if I am just not good at writing? It created a negative feeling of being a person of color. I just wanted to blend in and be treated like everyone else. As a PhD, I am constantly working harder because I know they are going to point out that English is my second language. I hate the association that when I suck, it is because I am an ESL learner." Pang Tao Moua

Pang Tao Moua, who is a PhD candidate and the first in her family to attend college, also had a completely different approach to the concerns regarding her English skills, which was for me really special to listen to and gave me a lot to think about. I had to ask myself some hard questions about the weight of my perception and approach to how I responded to comments, tones, and behaviors that made me feel assaulted.

> "I was the only minority student in my undergraduate program. I even changed my name to Paige because I was so tired of correcting the faculty and students repeating my name. Even though I was lonely, I saw it as a learning opportunity for the faculty and my classmates. I wanted to teach them about what it was like for me to navigate life being a minority student. I took it in a positive way. Because I was different, I often got to know the professors more, and they were very open to getting to know me. I taught them things, especially in phonetics. Oh! Phonetics was a hard class for me as Hmong is a tonal language."

Pang's testimonial was a big reality check moment for me, not because we both struggled in phonetics class, but I asked myself if I could have had a different attitude as I navigated my own barriers while pursuing my education. Could my attitude be the only factor why we had such different outlooks? Were the faculty in her university more open to these types of conversations and learning experiences? I don't know, but she sure brings a fresh air of positivity to this conversation.

I honor it.

Reflection Questions:

- What about your university experience do you think most contributed to a feeling of isolation?
- What contributed the most to a feeling of belonging?

Barbara Fernandes

Chapter 5:

Finding and Recognizing Your Support Network Elsewhere

"Giving connects two people, the giver and the receiver, and this connection gives birth to a new sense of belonging."
Deepak Chopra

In my mind, everyone who belongs to a minority group has at some point participated in the MSLP program. Unfortunately, that's just not realistic. So, girl, you and I gotta find a way for you to find your support network. Think of this support network as your family in the profession. They can come into your life in so many different forms. You may still not be convinced that you need a support network, or you may feel overwhelmed by the idea of looking for one. I will be honest with you, as an introvert myself, I rarely actually sought a support system for myself and failed at embracing it when it didn't feel organic. My support network just kinda fell on my lap, and I am eternally grateful for it. You know the joke? *How do introverts make friends? They don't. They wait for people to come to them.* It is okay if that's what happens for you too, but I want you to at least be much more conscious than I was about two things:

First, I want you to recognize the people who are already in your life who are serving as your support network. This could be your peers, your colleagues, a professor, a mentor, or a group of random strangers made friends from an online community. This recognition is a two-way process. You need to recognize it in your head, but you also need to, if you can, voice it out loud to the individuals. You would be surprised at the power of gratitude. If people are there for you, recognize them. This is not some cheap gimmick. Gratitude elevates your soul. If you feel it, say it.

Second, start feeling open to allow people to come into your life. I know that when we are in a state of survival, the world seems like this giant fog. It could be when you are trying to earn your current degree, learning to navigate your new job or position, surviving the work culture, starting your business, or even just surviving managing your business. When we are in a state of survival, we become hyper focused. I know I am guilty of that. When we are in that state, we may accidentally close ourselves off to an existing support system.

During my undergraduate program, I had Dr. Boyd and my professor from the language and culture class. Neither of them was an SLP, though. They were people who I could go to for advice while navigating a system that was brand-new for me. Looking back, I know that the fact that they were both coming from a minority background may have made them more compelled to support me. I will never know that for sure. However, I have a feeling that my interactions with my minority professors were just as important for them as they were for me.

Also during my undergraduate program at Temple, I built connections with other international and Latinx students. Some of those Latinx students had already tried to apply for Temple's bilingual program, and their rejection was my rejection. They had shared with me their multiple attempts to be accepted, which was why I didn't even attempt it myself. The international student friends I made gave me yet another perspective. While not a single one of those international students was attempting to earn an undergraduate in speech, it made me feel like I was not alone. Both of these examples show that the support I found during my undergraduate degree, both from peers and mentors, came from outside the CSD department. Sometimes, you have to find support and belonging elsewhere. Just go find it!

Upon returning from that ASHA Convention, having participated in the MSLP program, it was time for me to resume my first semester toward my two-year program at TCU. Things were much better at TCU than at Temple University. Here, I was one of four students who were admitted to the Bilingual program. There were two other Latina students, and I was able to find support from a few professors within the CSD program. Progress!

A lot of the awareness I am sharing here comes from looking back and reflecting. I want you to be more conscious than I was back then and more aware of your surroundings, how they affect you, and what you can do to keep going. During this phase of my life, I was also drowning. The bilingual program itself was rigorous, and that's okay. How rigorous a program is or isn't is not something in question here. What I want to talk about is going through a rigorous program while feeling left behind by some of your professors and your peers. Going through a graduate program and feeling like you don't belong, that's the real pain.

During my graduate program, my peers, some of whom have become good friends, generally speaking, came from similar backgrounds. Several attended TCU or other Texas-based universities for their undergraduate degree. I attempted multiple times to fit in. If you have not yet felt the weight of trying to fit in when you clearly don't, please take a moment to check yourself right here; it does not have to be related to the SLP world. I have become very conscious about making people feel included. When I have a birthday party at my house for example, if most of my guests are Brazilians, and I have one or two people who are outsiders or new to the group, I often go the extra mile to make that person feel welcomed and accepted. I make a conscious effort to bring the "lone wolf" in because of my own experiences with lack of embrace. I was lucky that this time I had one peer who made me feel less lonely, Veronica De La Cruz, the girl who apparently looked like me enough that I was often called Veronica. She was also called Barbara. Vero introduced me to her other Latina friends and would go on to become one of my bridesmaids at my wedding. When people are alone, it is the responsibility of the majority group to create an environment of inclusion.

I am not saying that my peers at TCU were a group of mean girls in high school like I see in Hollywood movies (remember I didn't go to high school in the USA); my peers were friendly. However, despite the friendliness, the underlying feeling I felt every time my peers got together to study for an exam or shared a very special resource that they got from someone they knew from a previous class among themselves and never shared with me, was that I did not belong.

Being an international student also means leaving behind most of your support network. While many universities have an office dedicated to international students, being a CSD student meant that I was not walking around campus. I hardly ever had the time to visit anywhere on campus besides the CSD building, where all the classes and clinical supervision took place. The feelings of isolation and loneliness were soul crushing.

Lack of time and sleep, stress, and isolation were perfect ingredients for a storm that could have been fatal for me. When it was time to study for my final exams in order to complete the program, my peers formed study groups in which I was not included. Since I lived over one hour away and needed to focus on studying, I rented a room at a cheap motel nearby and studied alone for hours. The feelings of fear and anxiety pushed me to the edge. One night, I thought I was having a heart attack and drove myself to the nearest hospital. On my drive, I was sure that I was either going to die from a heart attack or from a car accident. The sad thing is that I might even have wished for it. As soon as I entered the emergency room, I told them, "I think I am having a heart attack—please help me." The doctors who tended to me told me that I was having a panic attack and medicated me.

I was prescribed medication for home after staying at the hospital for a few hours for observation. I drove myself back to the motel and continued to study. Just a few hours later, I showed up at TCU to take the first of my final exams. I spoke to my program chair, and he kindly told me that I could take it another day. I knew that delaying it a day or two would actually make my anxiety worse, so I sat down and took the exam that morning. I didn't speak to anyone else about the incident. I felt so alone.

As I share this, I think about my peers who might one day read this; I don't want them to feel bad or embarrassed. I probably never allowed myself to be vulnerable enough for them to see me either. Vulnerability is where connections are formed. People can only know our struggles when we begin to share them, which is something that I was too afraid to do. As my peers appeared to have this strong bond among themselves, how could they ever relate to being alone? That's what I thought. Besides, being vulnerable when you can hardly keep yourself together seems like something too dangerous to get into. I was constantly in "Get your shit together, girl" mode.

I did have professors, such as Ms. Payne, my clinical supervisor for the bilingual program, and Dr. Ryan, the department chair who has since passed away, who were extremely supportive and understanding of my needs as an international student. Dr. Aker always gave me this feeling that she saw my potential behind my many inadequacies with my English skills. Following the pattern, the kindest person to me in that building was not an SLP, but Pat Brandt, the assistant to the chair of the department. Unfortunately, that support was only enough to keep me surviving.

A lot had happened to me prior to that nearly fatal drive to the emergency room. In my second semester at TCU, my father, who was battling cancer, was hospitalized. A call from my aunt told me it was time for me to come home. He passed away the day after I arrived. That loss was the most devastating blow to my life. Someone who already felt lonely was now even lonelier in the world. I was already struggling to survive the program before that loss. Things became even more difficult after it. However, I was not about to give up; in fact, his loss was a reminder of his sacrifices for my education. To add insult to injury, that spring, I also got into a major car accident on my way home from TCU. My car was totaled, and I suffered significant damage to my neck and back. I was prescribed potent narcotics to deal with my pain, which made it hard to keep up in class. That spring I was grieving my father while under the effects of narcotics. Attending classes just seemed impossible. Things sucked, but by then I was becoming a pro at bottling up all my pain and feelings and doing whatever it took to survive.

Eventually, I realized that I still had to complete my summer internships and two full semesters in order to wrap up my program and I could not keep going as I was. My father's loss was also a reminder of the fragility of life. I needed a break from school; I needed to heal; I needed to get back to a place in which hard exams were the only thing I had to handle.

I needed time away; I needed time on my own with my own thoughts and freedom to cry. When I was a child, my father used to tell me that I would travel to Greece one day. When I see the photos of my neighborhood and think of my family's economic conditions, I have no idea how my father could even let me believe in such a dream. When he passed, I needed to make it to Greece, but I knew my program would be unlikely to let me sit out my externships. As you know by now, I am the queen of clever ideas. I asked my program chair, Dr. Ryan, if I could postpone my summer externships and instead travel to Europe and investigate bilingualism there. I will never know if he bought my excuse for justifying my need for a break or if it was apparent that I needed a break; either way, he accepted. The bottom line is that I was allowed to complete my externship hours after my final semester in order to complete my mandatory placements. So I left, alone for the summer, with a ticket for unlimited train trips throughout Europe. Officially, I was on a quest to learn how Europe provided bilingual services, given their close geographical locations and large, diverse bilingual/bicultural populations. Unofficially, I was looking for healing. In the end, I accomplished both missions.

Reflection Question: Think about the people in your life right now. Who is part of your professional support system?

Chapter 6:

Be Uniquely You;
You Don't Have to Fit In

"When you are content to be simply yourself and don't compare or compete, everyone will respect you." Lao Tzu, Tao Te Ching

When you discover and believe deep in your soul that one of your superpowers is the fact that you have a unique point of view, things start to shift. Let's think about this: who would want to be just like everyone else? Not even my twin nieces do. I thought I did, and you may still think you do. However, once I realized that I was the only one who had the guts to postpone my graduation, buy a plane ticket to Europe, and spend three months roaming free on my own without a lot of money or planning, I knew I was unique. I think at that moment I started to believe that being uniquely me was pretty awesome. In fact, I believe that the fact that I had moved to a new country and left all the things I knew behind just three years prior is exactly what gave me this brand-new power to feel unique.

The fact is, I was feeling like being a Latina immigrant, who talked with a non-native accent and made a few too many errors with her prepositions (I still hate English prepositions) was becoming the most defining characteristic about me (especially in a college where professors would often call me by the name of the other Latina student in my class and vice versa). I was starting to forget that there was much more that made me who I am. I am an extremely adventurous and creative person who loves taking risks and who has already found unique solutions to overcome moments of past challenges. If I had not taken the chance to participate in that exchange student program, I would probably still be in Brazil, just like all my peers who did not take that risk. Embracing being uniquely me led to my very own uniquely-crafted path. Trust me, it is much easier to see what makes you unique as something to feel ashamed of when you are surrounded by people who are making you feel that way. Like Pang shared, I often wanted to blend in with everyone else in my cohort. Creating some distance between me and them at that time by traveling seemed like a wonderful idea. So I packed my bags and headed to Europe.

During my three months in Europe, I met with over fifteen speech-language pathologists in several countries, from the Czech Republic all the way to Portugal. Each of those clinicians was facing their own set of struggles and finding unique solutions to support the communication needs of a linguistically diverse community. It was brilliant, sis! I had previously arranged some of these meetings, and others I arranged while on the trip itself, all thanks to the beauty of the internet and emails. I will share some of the highlights.

One of the most memorable moments for me was meeting an American SLP named Pati Allen, who worked at a hospital near the London International Airport. She showed me around the hospital and shared with me that she was treating individuals who, combined, spoke more than twenty languages. Given the location of the hospital she worked at, that was the place where anyone arriving from the many flights around the world would be brought if they had medical issues during the flight. Many of the patients on her caseload were in-flight stroke victims. Can you imagine how clever you would have to be to evaluate almost a different language each day? When we made it to her office, she showed me her bookcase filled with different versions of Rosetta Stone software that she was using in conjunction with family support as a tool to help her assess the language skills of these patients in their native language. Brilliant!

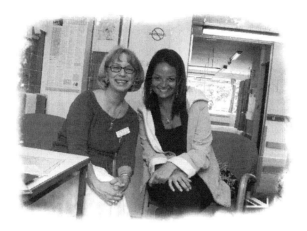

I traveled north in England to Manchester to meet with an SLT, Dr. Carol Stow, owner of a clinic that primarily treats the children of Indian immigrants. She had an incredible setup with three assistants, each of whom spoke a different language and dialect. This was the first time that I saw a clinician pay close attention to being culturally sensitive and responsible. She had dolls made that were culturally appropriate for her clients. Back in 2007, this was not a concept I had been exposed to or that was discussed much. They had even made custom traditional Indian clothes for the Barbie dolls. This was the first time that I was introduced to the importance of representation in the toys and dolls we use in therapy.

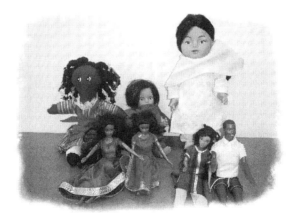

During my time in the Czech Republic, I got on a bus across town to try to find another SLP at a hospital. As soon as I arrived at the hospital, it was clear that I did not speak any of the languages that any of the staff spoke. While I had exchanged emails with this SLP to set up that meeting, this was 2007, and I didn't have a phone with access to the internet to contact her. Eventually, I did find her, and she didn't speak any English, Spanish, or Portuguese. So we went into her office and took turns using Google Translate to chat.

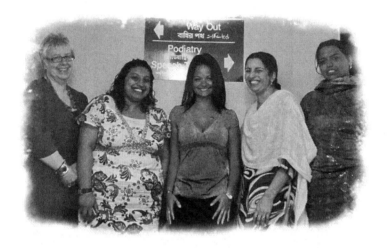

I could tell you hundreds of stories about the many SLPs I met on this adventure, the friends I made, and the nights I slept at airports, bus stations, kitchens, or on the balconies of complete strangers while couchsurfing. Couchsurfing was a thing prior to Airbnb; you could be hosted by random strangers willing to let travelers stay at their houses for free. Most days, I didn't have enough in my budget to eat two meals a day, so I relied on my host offering me a free breakfast, and then I would buy myself one meal out on the streets during my explorations. I made a lot of new friends in the hosts I met—some of which were immigrants to the country they were currently living in themselves. However, the lesson I want you to take from this is that none of my peers at TCU had the courage, the desire, or the spirit to embark on this adventure except me. I even invited a couple of them. They all said that I was crazy! And that's fine. They have their own unique talents, skills, and desires that make them who they are. But that experience became another pivotal moment in which I found a creative solution to overcome my struggles that led to even more lessons and growth. Through this, I was able to fulfill my dream to visit Greece and the Greek islands that my father said I would one day set foot on. I sat alone and watched the sunset, cried, and honored my father and the person I had become. On a lighter note: I even went to a wedding on a Greek island of a famous couple I never met before! Oh, the stories my kids will hear one day.

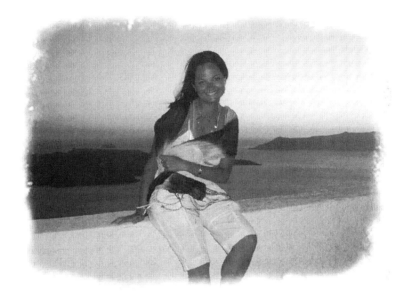

Once again, I returned home from that experience one step closer to owning up to my unique abilities. You don't have to travel to Europe and stay in random people's homes in order to find yourself and your unique abilities. What you need to do is start looking for and being proud of your unique abilities so that you can utilize them to take whatever road you choose for yourself. Not Barbara's road, your OWN. When I came back from that experience, I wrote my first article to the ASHA Leader as a student. But most importantly, when I returned, I felt like I had done something powerful not only at a personal level but also at a professional level. I was ready to own up to being a trilingual speech-language pathologist. I returned ready to take on my last year in graduate school.

Feeling much more confident about what I was bringing to the table, I was recruited for my first position as an SLP by a public school in the Dallas area before most of my peers, before even graduating. That happened because I was trilingual, and in the district where I got my first job, over 70% of the students identified themselves as coming from Hispanic heritage. I was able to advocate for a bilingual stipend for SLPs, which was not in place yet.

One of my favorite books that I read over ten years ago is *Outliers: The Story of Success* by Malcolm Gladwell—a reading I highly recommend. Gladwell talks about our need to pay attention to where successful people come from, their background and their experiences. I know that my unique experiences are exactly the reason why I thrive today.

When I started working for Irving ISD as a Clinical Fellowship Year (CFY), while being the only bilingual SLP in the entire district, it felt like I was stepping up yet again in finding a network of individuals who were also coming from a diverse background. Given the demographics of the district, I found myself interacting with several Latinx professionals, which was extremely refreshing. I no longer felt the need to hide the imperfect parts of me now that I was surrounded by professionals that included me in their lunch and occasional happy hour. My monolingual English-speaking peers called me to ask my advice on the bilingual students they were serving. My linguist skill was finally becoming one of my superpowers.

Regardless of how fast the demographics in the USA are still changing, not all of us will land in a region where we end up working with a population of clients that help us see the value that our background brings to the table. So, as much as I would like to tell you to move to someplace where your linguistic and/or racial/ethnic background is valued, honored, and respected, you shouldn't have to uproot your family and all that your full life offers in order to have that component. Let me be clear here, people don't have to look like you to value what you bring to the table. However, I will also tell you that spending eight hours a day surrounded by people who not only don't value what your background adds but actually put you down for it is soul crushing. The energy that it takes to try to blend in or hide the beautiful parts of you that they don't like leaves you empty and unable to be the amazing SLP you can be for yourself and for your clients.

"Embrace your uniqueness as early in your career as possible. Your rich cultural heritage is like a fingerprint that no one else has which makes your perspective that much more valuable. Your life experience shapes the way you interact with clients and colleagues, how you make clinical decisions, and how you create your future. Identify and love what makes you—you." Mai Ling Chan

As you keep reading, I will have some ideas on building a support network to get you started in your healing and growth path.

Reflection Question: What characteristics set you apart from your peers at school or at your workplace that you can utilize today to make moves?

Barbara Fernandes

Chapter 7:

Conflicts Within and Belonging

"I feel lost and confused, but happy and certain. I am like a ball of tangled yarn. The parts that are untangled are available, usable; the rest is a mess, useless until it is untied. That mess feels endless and at most times unyielding." Astrid Lee Miles, *Recovering is an Art*

As I write about many difficult subjects, it is also important for me to share that even though I am breaking down thoughts and ideas in different chapters, a lot of life does not happen in a continuum. I don't feel happy or sad all day every day; many days are filled with many conflicting emotions as we go through our lives. The same happened with the experiences I had in life. That's why I can feel grateful for an experience that actually led me to meet trauma. Sounds conflicting, right?

I know it is difficult to imagine, but back home I used to belong to the majority group. I was not "Latina," I just was. I had a family, a roof over my head, and I managed to attend one of the most prestigious public colleges in Brazil. I was an incredible communicator and had an awesome social life. As soon as I moved to the United States, I became a Latina labeled with a communication disorder, with whatever connotations that may have had at any given moment with whomever I interacted with. That shift was brutal. While immigrating to the US was a definite upgrade for my professional career, it was a major downgrade for my place in the world. That steep contrast was conflicting.

For years on end, I put a giant lid on the sadness of this transition because I was very aware of my privilege as an international student. But now, the more self-aware version of myself knows that it is also possible to feel the gratitude of privilege and the sadness for the immigrant status handicap at the same time. I felt, and still feel, incredibly privileged to be one in a million Brazilians who had the opportunity to move to the US in a position to continue to pursue my career of choice and arrive in this country through education with a sponsored J-1 visa. That's a big privilege, my friends! But it is also like having a million dollars in the bank but no one to share it with. Most of the Brazilian women I know today are lawyers, architects, teachers, and designers in Brazil, but when they immigrated to the United States they had to abandon that part of themselves and reinvent their lives. I am privileged to have been able to continue to follow the profession I chose as a seventeen-year-old even after immigrating. However, in feeling that privilege, I could never allow myself to acknowledge the pain and suffering caused by staying in the field.

To make the emotions even more complicated, as I mentioned earlier, my family and friends at home bragged about my accomplishments and how I was studying abroad. Many of my Brazilian peers, especially the ones from my community, would have given anything to be in my shoes. Little did they know, I had become the smallest fish in the ocean trying to swim with sharks ready to snap me out of the water. They had no idea about how isolated I had become, how much smaller people made me feel, or how that lighthearted person they once knew was driving herself to the emergency room alone in the middle of the night. I never shared any of this with them.

Many of us who come from families in which we are the first to go to college, buy a home, travel out of the country, or break other glass ceilings feel the pressure to keep up with the appearance that we are doing great. However, that does not invalidate the feelings that we are struggling within just to keep going. Just as gratitude can still exist while you struggle, disappointment, frustration, and trauma still happen while others see you living your best life. I can feel gratitude for having received a full ride at TCU while still acknowledging the scars that it left me with.

"My immigrant journey shaped my career, forcing me to make many plans—A, B, C, all the way until plan Z. I was always so fearful of having to leave the country that I tried really hard to brush things off and not let anything weigh on me too much. I guess I used the lens of 'I just can't be that sensitive' or 'I'm just reading into it and surely they didn't mean it in a racist manner.' So in many ways, I feel like I cushioned myself from the 'hurt' and maybe over time even became oblivious to it. Maybe in some ways I actually failed my fellow minority SLPs because I lived a life of privilege within the bubble I built for myself. There were several times when I didn't get an acute care position in my organization and was stuck in outpatient. I felt a lot of frustration, but I can't say I stopped to think about whether it was because of my race or ethnicity. I think that defense mechanism made me brush it off, like Teflon, versus have it stick like Velcro. So maybe that's a lesson in itself . . . too much Teflon isn't that great either." Ramya Kumar

These conflicting feelings were not only mine, or Ramya's, or unique to the immigrant community. During a vulnerable chat with Enjoli Richardson, an African American and Texas native, SLP, and PhD candidate at The University of Texas at Austin (UT Austin) at the time, she shared her feelings of conflict: being the one who was thriving from her community and a source of pride for her family, and not feeling worthy of being the one Black face within her cohort or that she had actually earned that spot in the sunlight. Enjoli, who grew up in a single-parent household and, like me, is the only one in her family to go to college, said, "We know in our heads that we belong here, but I still don't feel it in my heart that I am where I am supposed to be."

As we chatted for an hour, I could feel her; we empathized on so many levels. We also talked about our feelings of lack of true belonging, a feeling I experience in many places. She shared that when she goes home, she no longer quite fits in anymore as people can't relate to her struggles in academia. Yet as the only Black woman in her work cohort, she does not see faces or even cultural behaviors that resemble her own. She can't quite shake the feeling of not belonging in a majority white community. My experiences are the same; when I go back home, I have become too American, yet when I am in America, I am just not American enough.

There are also internal emotional conflicts I experience as a speech-language pathologist with an accent. I do understand the importance of being intelligible and the power of intelligibility in being an effective communicator. I longed to get back to the state in which people enjoyed hearing me talk. At the same time, I am aware that the listener also contributes to how intelligibly I am perceived. My husband often jokes with me that I am fluent in "globish," a totally made-up word we use to represent a global version of English I speak when I travel. He is impressed by how well I understand anyone's attempt to communicate with me abroad, regardless of their English level. I also naturally adjust my vocabulary and syntax to the listener to make sure I make myself understood and we can communicate as equals.

The less contact and interactions people have with people who speak with a non-native accent, the less they will understand our accented speech; however, somehow the burden always lies on me, not on the listener. My colleague Dr. Yao Du also shared her conflicts on this subject:

"As an international student, instead of choosing to go through the process of reducing my Chinese accent, I decided to take an active role in the 'driver's seat' and experienced being an accent reduction clinician. This was an unconscious decision, and I think I chose this path because back then, I wanted to learn how accent modification therapy worked, but I didn't want to lose my Chinese accent, which is an important part of my identity. Now as a professional, I learned that a lot of my bilingual Mandarin-English speaking SLP colleagues have had accent modification experiences while learning to become an SLP. Most of them were told to have their accent 'reduced' in order to become 'more professional' in this field. Cultural and linguistic diversity is one of the primary reasons that I am drawn to this field. However, with the rise of the #StopAsianHate movement during the COVID-19 pandemic, I also started to wonder: Did I contribute to systemic racism by providing accent modification services that privileges "Standard American English" as the gold standard? Did I do more harm than good to these clients? No one has the right answers for this." Yao Du, PhD, CCC-SLP

In the last few years, there has been a push for acceptance of neurodiversity and educating neurotypical individuals to be more understanding of everyone's individuality in their communication styles and behaviors. The push from autistic adults to be accepted as they are, such as how they might avoid eye contact and not necessarily be interested in looking neurotypical, has been a powerful movement from within the autistic community. As a mother of a child with autism, I have similar conflicts of balancing supporting my child's social skills, while at the same time educating his teachers on being more understanding, respectful and accepting of him as a whole child without forcing him to function as neurotypical children in all aspects. The autistic community wants neurotypicals to at least share the responsibility of having positive interactions with them. It is unfair to place the entire responsibility to adapt the communication style solely on the side of the autistic individual. I want the same thing to happen with accented speech.

While I have noticed a significant increase of accented speech on television, I am not seeing the same level of communication responsibility in our field placed on listeners to become more familiar with accented speech. I am also not seeing British, Irish, or Australian SLPs being forced to sound more "American." If the ultimate goal is to sound "American," this burden should apply to all non-American sounding accents, instead of the ones some deem to be "less valuable" accents. If we are promoting diversity, shouldn't our profession be training SLPs to be more prepared to understand foreign accented speech?

We wouldn't want everyone to look the same, so why do we push for everyone to sound the same?

Michelle Hernandez, an SLP and PhD candidate at the University of Houston, shared with me the moment she became aware of her cultural and linguistic differences. Michelle, who was born and raised in New York, is the daughter of Dominican parents. She talked to me about how she didn't realize how unique her diverse undergraduate experience was at Stony Brook University until she attended Buffalo State University for her master's program. There was a drastic shift in the feeling of belonging between her undergraduate and graduate program journey.

"During the first semester in my master's program, I was assigned a fluency evaluation practice case with two of my peers. While we were debriefing the results of the evaluation, one of my white male peers transcribed on a piece of paper in phonetics the word "ask" and asked me to say it out loud. I pronounced /aks/, which is how I grew up saying it. The word "ask" was in one of the prompts on the OWLS. Then he proceeded to correct my pronunciation, saying that both he and the client had trouble understanding me. Until that moment, in my entire life, nobody had made me aware of my dialect at all. I never thought I spoke any differently from anyone else because I come from a community where everyone talked like me. I was so upset that I started to cry. Things got worse when I spoke up about it with my cohort and more students started to say that they had trouble understanding me too." Michelle Hernandez, Dominican American SLP from NY

As I sat in my living room across the country, listening to Michelle's story, my heart ached for her. Her story exemplifies the obvious need to educate students beyond cultural competency for the clients we serve, but also the need for cultural sensitivity toward our bicultural colleagues. It is clear that carryover from one group to the other is not happening there.

Michelle continued, "Then one of the white girls asked, 'Aren't you Mexican? You make tacos?' I answered, 'No, I am not Mexican. I'm Dominican. I don't make tacos. I can, though. Just as much as I make pasta, and you aren't asking if I am Italian.' Then a second white girl asked, 'Why are you so offended?! We just brought up how you couldn't say one word.' So I answered how they were making fun of my accent as a whole, not just one word. During my program, I often heard questions like, 'Michelle, how do your parents work if they only speak Spanish?' I felt singled out often, not for anything positive, just because I was different." Michelle Hernandez, Dominican American SLP from NY

Despite the fact that all of Michelle's peers came from different states, they could find enough unity to single her out. We can't find belonging in places where we are made to feel inferior to the others in a group. Graduate school is hard as it is, but when our sense of worth is taken during this process, it can be debilitating. Obviously Michelle's peers had not yet had many interactions with immigrants or first generation Latinx, and their lack of ability to understand Michelle placed a burden on her. Michelle's peers never asked themselves how their inability to understand her might be coming from their own deficits of interactions with those with linguistic differences. Through the process of becoming an SLP, Michelle lost her sense of belonging in the very country she was born in. This is a price much higher than tuition.

Reflection Question: Can you think of conflicting feelings that you may have now that you need to acknowledge when it comes to your journey as an SLP thus far?

Barbara Fernandes

Chapter 8:

Surviving at Our Workplace

"I understood 'microaggressions' to mean 'little bullshit acts of racism.'" Gabby Rivera, *Juliet Takes a Breath*

I have realized that I come from a place of privilege when it comes to experiencing biases as an SLP at my workplace. I believe that happened in part because I was fortunate enough to live in a geographical area in which my language skills, as someone who spoke Spanish, were extremely valuable. Also, early in my career, I was working mostly with other Latinx or international professionals. Shortly after, I started my business, and I will discuss the impact of these types of interactions on me in future chapters. However, as my friend DM expressed clearly, it wasn't until recently that I started to be able to identify and acknowledge specific acts throughout my career:

"I look back on a lot of situations, and I realize that I didn't know what a microaggression was back then. I'd never heard that before. I didn't want to ruffle feathers. I didn't want to stand out for THAT, although I liked to stand out. I liked to stand out in terms of my ability to give presentations and in terms of my ability to shine academically, but I didn't want to be the one that was complaining about racism or sexism or any other -ism. I didn't want to be the one complaining. But you know what, it's okay. It's okay to say that things are not okay." DM

We often shake off short moments of discomfort that can have an impact on us, until the combination of all the moments starts to dawn on us.

"My experience in the field of CSD has been unique. I am Black, a first generation college student, and differently abled due to having a chronic illness that impacts my mobility. My undergrad experience was one that did not support my diversity adequately. I didn't feel supported, but I cannot identify true moments of bias and discrimination until I began working. I began working as a Rehab Director early in my career and wore a white lab coat every day. Yet I was never mistaken for the doctor. I was mistaken for the CNA often, and patients often assumed the one male on my staff was my boss. Working in rural NC, I was often questioned about my education and where I went to school or how I got my job. I was even called "that little colored girl" twice. If anything, these experiences made me more assertive. I learned I had to speak up for myself, educate people, and command respect. Once patients saw the progress they were making toward their goal while working with me or my ability to advocate for their family members, they were often so thankful, but I always wondered if I had not been Black, would I have been questioned about my education, mistaken for a CNA, or not recognized as the Director?" Jamila Perry Harley

Jamila's account of never being mistaken for someone in a position of considered status in our field reminded me of my own account of confusion from another SLP.

Some time ago, I was presenting at the CSHA Convention, and I was looking for the room I was presenting in ahead of time to check for their technology compatibility with my iPad. I saw a badge of someone who could assist me in finding the room. She was the chair of the CSHA Convention that year, so I approached to ask where the room was. She quickly dismissed me. "We only let presenters in the room right now." She was clearly surprised to learn I was a presenter myself. Someone who looked or sounded like me could actually be a speaker? Should I have spent hours dwelling on that encounter? Absolutely not! That's what happened. Overthinking is the worst. Maybe I should have learned from Ramya's book and let that slide like Teflon.

Giving presentations can reveal different types of microaggression. I am often looked at under a microscope for whatever possible word I might mispronounce at a given moment. Yet again, I know I am not alone:

"There was the colleague who told me following a presentation to thousands that I mispronounced a word." Phung Palafox

Have you ever seen Phuong speak? I have, and you should. Phuong writes and speaks like an SLP poet. Why would one of our colleagues decide to focus on her pronunciation of one single word among the thousands she likely spoke during that presentation. Can you hear me scream WHYYYYYY???????

The same bullshit happens with our very own American-born Black SLPs too. Ebony Green had her own fair share of experiences with people being surprised about how "articulate" she was upon meeting her in person and getting to see what she looked like. She decided to share this story with us.

"In August 2014, I started a new job as an SLPA at a charter school in Arizona. I was ecstatic to be at a new school in a beautiful building. This was my second SLPA job, and I'd heard great things about this particular school. Ever since my first day, the teachers were all nice, and the principal was nice to me too. It seemed like the perfect job, and everyone made me feel so welcome.

Sadly, my reality changed when I met the Special Education Director for the first time a couple of weeks later. She and I had exchanged emails a few times after I started working at this new school, and she seemed like a nice, approachable person, despite how busy she must have been. One day she sent me a calendar invite to meet in person. She said she would be at my campus to meet some of the special education teachers and wanted to meet me as well.

The next day, I arrived at school and as soon as I sat down at my desk, a woman approached me and said, 'Hi, I'm Lisa.' I shook her hand and said, 'Hi Lisa, I'm Ebony.' The next thing that came out of Lisa's mouth still haunts me to this day, and probably will for the rest of my life. She looked me in the eye and said, 'Oh, wow, who would've known that Ebony was actually . . . Ebony.' I felt numb. My face got hot. My heart started racing. I wanted to run away and hide. What did this woman just say? What the actual f? I could not believe she made such a racist, bigoted remark about me being a Black woman.

At that moment, I experienced so many emotions at once; however, I couldn't let her see me sweat. Who knew what stereotypes she already believed about Black people, and the last thing I wanted to do was perpetuate those stereotypes. I chuckled and said, 'Well, my last name is Green, so just imagine how surprised you would've been if I were Green too.' I later went home and told my husband and friends about the situation. I cursed Lisa out in my head, and I reevaluated my response and what I should have said. I gave myself a pep talk on my way to work every day about how qualified and skilled I was for my job and reminded myself that my students and colleagues were lucky to have me despite what someone else's preconceived racist notions about women of color were.

This experience is one that will always remind me that I am in the 8.5%. When I think about that day, not only do I get angry and a little embarrassed, but I also get energized to prove people like Lisa wrong. Since that day, it has been my mission to show the 'Lisas' out there that women who look like me are just as capable, intelligent, and competent as women with ivory skin. I AM EBONY, and I am Proud!"
Ebony Green

I am proud of how Ebony responded. I know that the Barbara of yesterday would have spent days wondering what had just happened, unable to give an answer on the spot. As the typical overthinker, I would have rehearsed the answer I would never give in my head over and over again. The comment that Ebony had to respond to came from within our field, and it did not happen in the 1800s.

At times, as SLPs who look different from our own clients, even as second-generation Americans, we still experience the impact of being treated as outsiders, which is what my colleague Mai Ling Chan experienced.

"I have shared this story of prejudice several times, and it still makes me shake my head thinking about it. I am American, born in Hackensack, NJ, and have a hint of a NJ accent when I speak. My mom, also born in NJ, is Colombian, and my father, Chinese from Hong Kong, earned his American citizenship fighting in the Vietnam War. My experiences with prejudice have occurred throughout my life, but this one incident is a perfect example of judgment without cause. It occurred while working in a very reputable hospital in a primarily Caucasian geriatric community providing in-patient acute care. It was nearing the Christmas holiday, and the nurse's station was already festively decorated with garland and stockings and plenty of homemade cookies and snacks filled the break room for our staff. I entered a new patient's room while he was sitting upright in bed with his spouse at his bedside. As per my typical routine, I announced myself and requested permission to enter, 'Hi Mr. (last name), I'm Mai Ling Chan, the speech pathologist, may I come in?' He responded 'Sure!' in a friendly tone, and I crossed the room to his bed. Already informally assessing his cognition and speech, I decided to open the session with organic conversation using a non-denominational, open-ended question, 'Will you be celebrating the upcoming holiday?' to which he responded, 'Yep. Kids are flying in for Christmas, and Mom here is going to start cooking soon. I need to get home in time for the festivities.' 'Sounds wonderful!' I replied. And then he said, 'What do they do in YOUR country?'" Mai Ling Chan

I had honestly not considered including the experiences of minority SLPs with our clients, partly because I am sure that many of us have enough stories to share in that department that it could become its own book. My primary goal with this book was to initiate discussions around the struggles that minority SLPs have with our peers during our education and training, our colleagues at the workplace, and in our profession as a whole. Mai Ling's story, though, serves as a reminder to all of us that at times, our professional experiences are bombarded with messages that we are outsiders, and/or we do not belong. I, fortunately, have not had much to share in that arena. I also have hope that the increased representation of diverse casts on TV will help our society advance in this aspect; I have hope that we will all soon have more and more positive and inspirational stories to share about our encounters with the people we have dedicated our professional lives to support.

Barbara Fernandes

As I close this section of the book, you have read a lot about me and the many SLPs who shared their stories of survival. Now it is time to hear us thrive!

Part Two: **Thriving**

"The way to thrive is to help others thrive; the way to flourish is to help others flourish; the way to fulfill yourself is to spend yourself."
Cornelius Plantinga

While this book is divided into three main sections, I do not want you to imagine that once I earned my master's degree all I did was thrive. No, ma'am. That's far from my reality. I had many days in which I was barely surviving, even this year. However, I can say that I am now in a general state of thriving, with some survival mode days, as opposed to spending long periods of time feeling that I can hardly keep my head above water. Throughout this section, you will read about how the risk taking stakes got higher, how I was still afraid, and how there were days that I didn't think I could go on. That master's degree did not shield me from being reminded of what I sound like and where I come from, but slowly I became more equipped to handle the blows and surprises when they came.

Earning a professional diploma puts us in the driver's seat of our decisions. The field of speech pathology is vast and offers a lot of opportunities for us to discover what brings us joy. However, the process of finding joy requires us to examine a lot of our preconceived notions about what an SLP can do. Ultimately, we are only limited by our capacity to imagine, our code of ethics, and the law. We don't have to follow an existing path.

When I applied for my master's program, I was eager to attend a program that had emphasis on bilingualism. My experience as a foreigner who had just learned two new languages two years prior to that propelled me to think that this was my calling. You might be surprised to know that during my undergraduate program in Brazil, my dream was to be an SLP who specialized in voice. My undergraduate thesis was on singing voice. My hometown was the mecca of music in Brazil. I had this vision that one day I would be working with famous singers from my country, but life opened different doors for me; all I had to do was to make decisions to lead me to the amazing life I get to experience today. I want you to experience the same joy that I have, that comes from the feeling that you are on vacation every single day because you love your occupation. However, in order to do that, I believe the first step is to increase your awareness of who you truly are.

My goal in this section of the book is to give you a glimpse of the key aspects I found to be essential to overcome the obstacles I shared in the first sections of this book. I will expose you to a unique perspective about thriving as a minority SLP. I will share how I carved my own unique job description despite the mountains I had to climb for it. My hope is that you feel inspired to go out there and craft your own job title, despite your personal mountains and setbacks, if that is what you wish.

Let's do this thing!

Chapter 9:

Gaining Self Awareness

"Self-awareness gives you the capacity to learn from your mistakes
as well as your successes. It enables you to keep growing."
Lawrence Bossidy

At the 2021 ASHA Convention, I attended a session by my good SLP friend, Tara Roehl. She reminded people in the room that if we assess our students' skills, and we spend a lot of time trying to figure out our students' strengths and weaknesses, we should also respect ourselves enough to spend some time asking ourselves the same questions. Do you know your superpowers? What is your kryptonite?

At some point in my life I became much more interested in reading self-help books. One of the things that I love the most about them is that even if I don't quite agree with the author, it helps me take a stand about *why* I don't agree, which leads to getting to know more about myself. Gaining awareness about who you are, your values, your background, and your flaws is, in my opinion, essential to thriving. Hopefully this book is doing that for you. You can read my words and decide which parts you identify with and which parts you disagree with. This exercise will, in and of itself, lead you to gain more awareness about yourself.

I have been looking in the mirror for a long time, but it was only in the last four years that I became obsessed with personality tests. I took my first one at the house of a friend whose husband is a psychologist. The test was called Personality Dimensions, which placed me in the orange category and it really opened my eyes to things I had never even thought about. From their website, "Personality Dimensions® is about understanding yourself and others so you can be more effective in your relationships, your work . . . your life." As soon as I came home, I started to post on my Instagram about how proud I was to be mostly an "Orange" personality with some "Green." From their result, my personality had the following strengths: trouble shooter, flexible, determined, spontaneous, risk-taker, creative, works well under pressure, multitasker, thinks outside the box, problem solver. Thanks to my orange personality I ride a motorcycle, play drums, and have an advanced scuba diving certification. The green side of me was where my innovation, logic, and independence comes from. Those are totally me!

There was so much power in being associated with those adjectives, and I want you to take time today to find your own adjectives. There are several online tests that you can take. One of my favorites, which is also free, is the 16 Personalities test (https://www.16personalities.com/free-personality-test). Go ahead, stop reading my words, and go take your test. Once you read the test results, one of the most important steps is reflecting on if you feel like they actually gave you the words that match what you already feel you are. If not, that's just as powerful because you can tell yourself why and why not.

My result on the 16 Personalities test came out as the *Advocate* personality, which explains a lot of what you have already read in this book and a lot that you are going to read in the following chapters. Even though this is the rarest of the sixteen types, many of my close SLP friends also had the same result. We are in the right field: advocating for individuals with communication disorders.

As I mentioned, there are a lot of other personality tests online. The ultimate goal, no matter which one you choose, is to make a conscientious effort to give vocabulary to your strengths and weaknesses. I wish I had been doing that much sooner in life. The more soul searching you do, the more powerful you become. If you are new to this, don't worry. Just get started taking control juggling the great and not so great things life throws at you.

During my Clinical Fellowship Year (CFY), I finally started to be recognized for being someone more than "the Brazilian student," or even more vaguely and inaccurately, the "Hispanic student." Brazilians are Latinx, but not Hispanic. Hispanics are individuals who speak Spanish. Brazil is in Latin America, but we are Portuguese speakers. I will confess that, as someone who has been surrounded by Hispanic friends and who loves speaking Spanish, I actually like it when people assume I am Hispanic. Nonetheless, Brazil and French Guiana natives, for example, are Latinx but not Hispanics.

My work colleagues recognized me as someone who cared for my students and someone who was dynamic, creative, and extremely efficient. Those were things that I also saw in myself. However, I still struggled navigating the special education system. As an immigrant who did not attend school in the US, I had no idea how basic things functioned within the US school system—from how many grades were in each grade level to the chain of command. I felt extremely self-conscious about the fact that I was still learning things that my American-born colleagues already knew. However, none of those things defined me anymore. I was adding to any team I joined, not only with my skills as a speech-language pathologist, but especially with my language skills. The table had finally flipped. Being trilingual was no longer a handicap; it was an advantage, and that, my friends, is a powerful fuel to confidence.

When I returned from my European adventure, I was more aware that my language learning skills were not within the average range. During my time in Italy, I was amazed at how knowing two Roman languages allowed me to understand some Italian. I realized that learning languages was another area that not only was I good at, but it brought me joy. So, I decided to learn a language that I have always loved to listen to music in: Arabic. I enrolled myself in Arabic class during my master's program. I took two semesters of Arabic at TCU. I also started using a language learning program called Pimsleur. Through Pimsleur, I learned some French and expanded my skills in Arabic as well. If you are an auditory learner like me, you can easily access Pimsleur language training on most online audio marketplaces. My multilingual skills became a huge asset during my first two years as an SLP in a highly diverse school district.

I quickly recognized that I also had a drive for problem solving. My happier days were the ones in which I traveled across campuses, evaluating students from diverse linguistic backgrounds. I loved the interactions I had with caregivers. I loved getting to be a problem solver. It is a role that changes each day and has many unexpected outcomes. That worked well with my personality. Eventually, I was spending more of my time as an evaluator than delivering therapy to students.

Exploring my strengths led me to another interest: after earning my master's degree, I enrolled at a community college to take photography classes. I had a ton of fun learning about visual composition and many other aesthetic aspects of photography, including how to properly frame images and see the photo before pressing the shutter. My love for learning and my risk-taking personality even had me ready for the lockdowns during the COVID-19 pandemic. I had experimented with cutting my own hair five years prior and have been doing it since. Nothing is as risky as cutting your own hair. LOL. I was probably the only person with wonderful haircuts throughout the pandemic. Laughing emoji face.

All jokes aside; do you see a pattern here? I have never stopped being a student. At first, it may seem that I was learning random, unnecessary skills. It seemed that way to me too, but whatever I learned has always helped me reach the next level. As a teen, I never thought I would make use of my website building skill. But it actually allowed me to attend an English school in Brazil. I had no idea why I needed to learn English, or what I would ever use it for, but it gave me a chance to at least consider applying for an exchange student program that eventually brought me to the USA. My photography skills also became an important piece of my life's puzzle.

I promise that the skills you learn, no matter how unrelated to speech therapy and communication disorders they may seem, can and should be integrated into your service delivery.

As soon as I signed the contract for my first job, my first purchase was the latest piece of technology that I had been dreaming about: the iPhone 3G. Yeah, it sounds lame several years later. Remember when I said I was about to switch my major just two years prior to this? I was going to go to an IT field. I love technology. I grew up playing video games, and I taught myself how to design websites. Technology brings me joy, and it has always been my hobby. Buying my very first iPhone brought me so much more than happiness. It was that one piece of technology that would transform me and an entire field.

Knowing yourself doesn't just involve knowing the parts of you that make you look good. It also involves knowing the parts of yourself that you can't showcase to everyone. As you look back, you may see that you have already found creative ways to handle those parts of yourself so they don't sabotage your dreams. I did this too.

When I started college in Brazil, I became very concerned about my inability to remember things, tend to others, and a myriad of other things that I thought were affecting my ability to function in college. I remember studying neurology at eighteen years old, and I was convinced that I had some sort of degenerative neurological condition. Around this time, I was diagnosed with attention deficit disorder (ADD). That diagnosis is part of a bigger umbrella of ADHD (attention deficit and hyperactivity disorder). Before this, I was overwhelmed by the idea that I might be dying. The ADD diagnosis was a wonderful explanation for why I was grounded more than any of my friends growing up for losing things or "playing like a boy." It also explained why I didn't even bother following instruction most of the time and preferred to study alone at night on my own at a much faster pace.

Now that I am more aware of how my brain works, I can look back and see how I had always found ways to accomplish goals through managing how my brain functions. Growing up in Brazil in a lively neighborhood in a small home, it was always impossible for me to study in the daytime. I could not function with the TV on, the neighbor's music, the dog barking, and all the other random noises everywhere. I found myself studying mostly at night on the kitchen table after everyone went to bed. I never associated much of how I operate in life, including my risk-taking behaviors, to ADHD until my husband decided to read a book on it recently, called *ADHD 2.0* by Edward M. Hallowell and John J. Ratey. He shared this quote with me:

"We (people with ADHD) lack an internal sense of the art of time. We define the laws of physics, and we change the nature of time in our minds. In our world we have a little awareness of the seconds ticking by—We only recognize two times, now and not now."

I have a sense of urgency in making things happen. I am not sure how much of my neurodiversity contributes to this. In my opinion, that's irrelevant because I choose to see myself as a whole person, not as one of my diagnoses. (I hope you are also doing this for yourself and your clients.) This urgency makes it so that when I decide that I want something, I can't dwell much on it. I have to get started. I put in a massive amount of energy to get it done in the shortest amount of time possible because I know that if I don't do it this way, it will drag on for too long, and my attention will shift toward the next shiny thing. When I decided that I was going to write this book, I opened Google Docs after an exhausting day at an ASHA Convention, and I started writing. I wrote every single day after, for I was determined to write this book in thirty days. As a mother of two kids under eight years old, my house is always noisy. In order to focus my attention on writing this, I am wearing headphones and listening to my favorite music as I type.

As a clinician who had the least crafty inclinations, technology became my lifeline. In my CF year, my clinical supervisor would often find me utilizing a variety of video games with the students I was servicing. I was obsessed with using *The Sims* for language therapy. If you are young, let me tell you that back in my day, if I wanted to utilize games as a therapy tool, I had to bring a CD-ROM to the office, install the game on a computer, and wait for the game to load (very slowly). I didn't let my poor craft skills hold me back from supporting my students with fun and engaging resources.

I sound like an old woman here. Girl, I am young. I'll stop speaking as if I'm old as soon as I tell you that I am from the age in which, if I wanted to create a visual support, I had to go to my school's library and check out the CD for running the support program; and I had to return it by the end of the day. There was no creative way around that, until I actually managed to create my own improved online resource creation platform.

By now, you know that I am a neuro-diverse, adventurous risk-taker, who loves learning languages and technology. The great thing about taking risks that keep paying off is that you will keep on taking more risks. I love that! A big part of thriving in anything in life is having some level of self-awareness, not only about who we are, but also about what kind of life we want for ourselves. Have you stopped to think about that?

Life happens fast for me. Since I moved to the US in 2004, I had finished an exchange student program, earned two degrees, learned two new languages, participated in two additional educational programs abroad, traveled to eighteen countries, got married, got my first job, and by January of 2009, I filed with the state of Texas to open my first business: Smarty Ears. All the events in this paragraph took place in four and a half years of my life.

I don't want you to think that when I filed for the formation of Smarty Ears I had it clear in my head. I had no idea what I was doing. I just figured, I love technology, and I am this kick-ass problem solver; so I am going to do this! Remember the book I mentioned earlier, *Outliers*? I feel like I was the right person, with the right skills and experiences, at the right time, who actually took a chance to take the very first step. It took me years doing business before I ever wrote my first business plan!

The idea for my business came from the fact that I was the only SLP I knew who was willing to let students use the most expensive piece of equipment in the room (with the exception of those very expensive, clunky AAC devices): my iPhone 3G. Apps for speech therapy didn't exist yet, but remember that up to that point I was pulling CD-ROMS from the library. Now, I had a device far superior to any computer, portable, and it was something that would respond to the kids' touch. This is the point in which I wanted to insert the mind blown emoji, but it has been twelve years now and touch technology no longer impresses you. Laughing emoji.

My students were all pre-K and kindergarten students. I was making significant progress, especially with my non-verbal students, simply by saving photos from Google onto my iPhone and letting them swipe the screen. I thought to myself: How does one go about making apps? I had no idea where to start.

So yeah, I had no business experience and no idea how to go about making an app. But if there is a will, there's a way. The awareness of what made me uniquely me began unlocking my superpowers, and this led me from no app to my first app, and then many more.

Reflection Question: What are some of the things that bring you joy today, and how could you integrate them in your service delivery to make it even more joyous to you and your clients?

Barbara Fernandes

Chapter 10:

Unlocking Your Superpower

"You are ok. You are, in fact, more than that! You are worthwhile! You are worth it! YOU are worthy! Even when you do not feel like it, you are! Be strong and courageous! We all have a different journey, and each journey is unique! Your journey is uniquely, beautifully YOURS! Embrace it!" Ashley Howard Nelson

The day that I decided to post an ad on Craigslist to hire a developer to implement my very first edtech idea, I had no clue how that was the first step to the life of my dreams. Craigslist is a place where you can post local ads to hire people for gigs, and I felt like I was not ready to employ anyone; I was still employed as an SLP at the public school.

I won't resort to my old lady words of, "You kids these days have so much more than I had when I started my business." These days you can hire freelancer developers on websites such as Upwork.com and Fiverr.com and give your next idea a go. Wink. Wink.

A few people applied to my job post, and the one person who caught my attention was a programmer who had a full-time job working for Verizon. We spoke on the phone and decided to meet in person at a Starbucks after our shifts at our full-time jobs. During our meeting, I explained to him that I wanted to create an app for iPhone for articulation. I had to explain what articulation meant. The descriptions probably sounded like this:

"I would like you to program an app for me where the therapist can add student names, then select that profile to start a session. The therapist should be able to select from a series of buttons; each would represent a sound. Then they can select from three options: initial, medial, or final. The activity is basically a way to sort these photos by their sound and the position in which these sounds appear. When we display the photos, the therapist should be able to click either a correct or incorrect button to represent if the child's production of the sound in that word was correct or not. The app should track and calculate the percentage of accuracy for each session and store that data over time for every time the therapist sees that child."

That was the birth of the very first app for speech therapy on the App Store. During that meeting, he told me that he would charge me US $4,000 to create that app for me if he could create it on a technology called PhoneGap. That total amount was more than what I was bringing home in a whole month as an SLP in public schools, but he told me I would pay him a certain amount for him to start, then the rest when the app was finalized. I agreed, and I went home to get started on my part of the work in order to bring that app to life.

In order to give him a visual idea of how the app should flow, I went to town on Microsoft Powerpoint. I envisioned all the screens and the behavior of each button. Then for a week straight, I would get home and come up with words for each of the sounds in each position. I licensed images from a copyright-free company. I worked through the night in order to have my word lists ready and the images to go with each word. My developer needed those before he could actually program the words into the app. I had to think of the name for the app and a logo to be used on the icon. By December of 2009, *Mobile Articulation Probes* was made available on the App Store under my company Smarty Ears, and it was sold at a one-time price of $29.99. That app no longer exists; it evolved into the most popular app I ever created, even making it to Apple's Best Selling: *Articulate Plus*.

In a matter of two to three months, I went from having an aha moment to having the first app for speech therapy actually for sale on the App Store. Having just read the previous chapter, this fast timeline may no longer surprise you. If you are a planner, someone who's organized, and who values stability, you are likely cringing. All you may have read was, "An SLP hires this dude from the internet, gives him money upfront to create an app that she has no idea if she will even make her money back on." The same story can sound completely different to different people. Taking risks and starting a business is not for everyone, and it is only one of the many paths that you have ahead of you to thrive within our field. I still keep in touch with that developer, mostly via Linkedin. He, who is also an immigrant, has since started his own business with brand-new hardware and software for renting work cabinet spaces.

I knew I was finally unlocking my superpower by continuing to take risks. As I shared in the previous chapter, getting to know yourself is the most significant step in thriving. When it comes to knowing yourself and finding the path in the field that is most likely to bring you joy, getting a feel for how our work environment will affect you is extremely valuable as well. Some of us are loners; some of us need the collaborative aspect to thrive. There is no best way. There is only the way and place that feels comfortable to you and aligns with your goals and who you are.

Often, we end up discovering the many things we don't like before we actually stumble upon a path that feels right.

Exactly a year ago, I was approached by a male, non-SLP entrepreneur in our industry with a proposal to merge my business with his. He was developing a telehealth platform, and given my collection of apps, it seemed like a perfect fit for a partnership. I was feeling overworked and burned out from running my businesses solo, and he had a track record of, more often than not, succeeding in his business ventures. This was the very first time that I entertained teaming up with someone else. We had a series of meetings, presentations, and discussions about what this relationship would look like. While it seemed like a possible financial opportunity, ultimately I told him I was not interested in pursuing it any further.

Lucky for me, he asked me one pivotal question:

"Would you rather be the sole owner of a x million dollar company, or the owner of a 10x million dollar company with partners?"

This was the exact moment it became clear in my head that the amount of money I was making was not the reason why I started or stayed in business—it was to live a comfortable life while being the boss of my time and decisions and supporting my colleagues by creating innovative technology that supports children and adults with communication disorders. That is what brings me joy.

Don't get me wrong, we all love the extra numbers in our bank account, and for some people, that's what drives them. That's perfectly okay. My businesses are not a hobby; they are highly profitable, and I care a lot about growing more each year. However, one of the key things in being primarily an "orange personality" type is freedom. Once I went back and looked at what brought me joy, I moved from a state of indecisiveness to a solid state of knowing who I was and why I woke up with so much joy each morning to fulfill my mission. That awareness was emboldened by exploring myself and giving words to what makes my heart do the happy dance.

Reflection Question: What are the top three adjectives that most drive your professional decisions in life?

Chapter 11:

All Comes at Once. Serendipity? Maybe.

"And, when you want something, all the universe conspires in helping you to achieve it." Paulo Coelho, *The Alchemist*

While I write this book, you might have gotten the idea that I am sitting somewhere calm and quiet and that I had all the time in the world to just sit and write. I have my son's eighth birthday party in five days, my kids were home last week during Thanksgiving break, I am selling a piece of land I bought, and I still have to run two businesses. My kitchen still needs to be cleaned, and I will have a day with a few meetings in between writing. Life did not stop so I could actually sit and write this book. That's not how life happens for anyone. We are often tempted to wait until life settles before taking on the next project. I urge you to stop doing that. What is the chapter of your life that you will be writing next?

The first page of this book was written while I was still attending the 2021 ASHA Convention, after a long day standing and talking to customers at the Smarty Ears booth, and after attending one of the many evening events. When I decided to start my businesses, I was still working at the public schools. I had evaluations to write, students to see, and therapy sessions to plan. For the first year of my business life, I was working in the public schools.

The fact that other events come into play at the same time that you are making your moves toward a life that aligns more closely to your strengths can either give you clarity or make you lose sight of what is important. For me, my work in the public schools gave me clarity and strength to take the next step: quit my full time job.

As my third year was starting, and as the only bilingual SLP in a large district in the diverse Dallas area, things shifted from, "Barbara, pick the fires you wanna put out," to "Barbara, we want you to handle all the fires." Over time, I started to feel the unfair distribution of workload. My monolingual English SLP colleagues in the pre-schools had a much smaller therapy caseload than I did. That extra bilingual stipend was starting to feel less and less worth the exhaustion and stress of being the only bilingual evaluator for three preschools, delivering therapy, and being part of the autism assessment team for the district.

As the next school year began in fall of 2010, the pressure I was under was really taking a toll on my mental health. I started to dread the process of waking up and going to work every morning. The only reason I was keeping up with my workload was because I was extremely efficient.

To make things worse, as someone who had attended every single ASHA Convention until then, I made plans to do so again in 2010. I asked my principal for time off to attend the convention, and he said that I had to take my sick days if I wanted to go. I wrote to the special education director, who gave me the same answer. I was now overworked at a school district that did not support my professional development needs and professional aspirations. Remember what I said in the previous chapter about us sometimes knowing what we don't want before actually stumbling onto what we do want? I knew that I wanted to work somewhere that wouldn't make me take a sick day to attend the ASHA Convention.

Fear not, sis, other life stories are also beginning to take shape because life did not stop, and all was happening at once. The seeds I planted a year ago were starting to transform into a beautiful tree. Meanwhile, what started as an idea, hiring a guy from Craigslist to create my first app, was now a collection of apps starting to take the shape of a real business. One year after releasing my first app, I had ten apps on the App Store.

I had no idea that releasing that first app was going to be any more than some extra vacation money. I love to travel! I remember doing the math in my head almost every day: "If I sell one app a day at $29.99, after Apple takes their 30% cut (go ahead and gasp here too), I could take home almost an extra $600 a month." That was exciting enough for me. The app that had hit the App Store in December of 2009 made back my investment by February of 2010. Around March, I had my very first booth at the Texas Speech and Hearing Convention (TSHA) in Fort Worth, Texas.

Bless my heart, as they say around here. I look at the pictures of my booth, and all I see are random pieces of laminated paper versions of my apps and a duck balloon from Party City. My booth's design left a lot to be desired, to say the least. I had no idea how to do a booth setup. A couple years ago, I was going through my company's photos on Facebook, and I was so embarrassed at how Smarty Ears' first booth looked that I deleted that photo. Today, I am no longer embarrassed; booth decoration is not one of my strengths and that's okay. I am proud of how far I have evolved in my ability to have a professional-looking booth at trade shows, despite my clear handicap in this area.

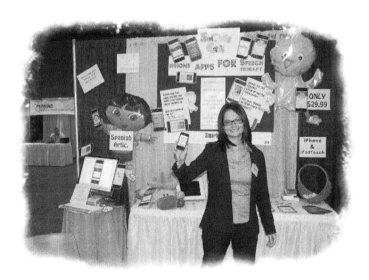

That's my first book at the TSHA Convention in March of 2010

Life does not stop just so you can start planting your seed. I was having panic attacks at my daytime job, but I was also generating just as much income on my side gig developing apps. Since I had just bought my first home, the thought of taking on a business full time, with all the uncertainty that comes with it, was terrifying. However, given my district's inflexibility in ensuring access to quality continuing professional education for its employees, by October of 2010, I gave my school district my resignation letter with a two weeks notice.

I did not have it in me to do the job to the best of my abilities any longer. I now had the freedom to not only attend, but to actually have my very first booth at the ASHA Convention. That second booth looked a lot better than the TSHA booth a few months prior. It was scary, but it was so exciting!

You may still be a student, or you may already have a family that depends on your ability to generate income. For me, the idea that I didn't know if I was actually selling apps at any given day was terrifying. While my husband had a job as a public school English teacher, we depended on both of our salaries to pay our bills. I had a student loan, a mortgage, car payments, and all the other adult life expenses, and I had just quit my stable income source, and most importantly my health insurance source. Remember how I said that when you thrive, it does not mean you don't still have survival mode moments too? This is exactly what I am talking about.

The fear of taking on my role as Smarty Ears CEO without a stable income stream led me to start working as an independent contractor evaluator for two companies in the Dallas area two to three days a week. I was able to land these contracts within a week from my last day as a full-time school clinician. As a trilingual SLP, there was a lot of demand from school districts and private practices to have me come in and evaluate students in their schools or homes. This transition time gave me the peace of mind of a more stable income stream, while giving me more flexibility and time to grow Smarty Ears. My own business was no longer a weekend or weeknights gig; I was able to dedicate two full days a week just for Smarty Ears. Don't get me wrong, I was still working nighttime too.

By now, I had gotten better at designing apps and icons, and I had a dedicated team of offshore developers. I had developed apps for articulation therapy, WH-questions, fluency tracking, verbs, a chronological age calculator, and even an app for voice. However, my best work was when I developed the *Articulation Assessment Toolkit*, which is to this day—more than a decade later—my best, most innovative work.

As you read about my breakdown at my full-time job, my embarrassment that my first booth looked like a hot mess, and my fears about making sure I could pay my bills, I want you to see that life was not pausing while I was taking steps. I didn't withdraw my booth because I knew I was not good at it. I kept moving forward. If you have gotten this far in my book, I know that you also have one million doubts about your ability to take the next step. I did too! I didn't take my steps without my many doubts. They were with me the whole time; they are still here.

As I sat in my ugly booth at the TSHA Convention, SLPs came to chat with me, curious about what I could possibly be exhibiting. You want to know what I heard the most from them that year?

"There is no way I will let my students play with the most expensive device I own. My iPhone is my baby."

They were right! It was a hard proposition for them. While they loved the idea that I was offering, to have thousands of pictures organized by their phonemes—the equivalent of hundreds of dollars in three dozen articulation flashcards boxes—the idea that a student would eventually destroy their personal equipment was stronger than that. At least at that particular point in time.

I realized that I was facing an uphill battle just to get my fellow clinicians to even begin to adopt the new technology. That was also the beginning of my journey as a blogger and a video podcaster called GeekSLP. If you are looking for some laughing time on my dime, go ahead and search for my 2010 videos on YouTube. You can find them by searching GeekSLP. You will find some great videos about the latest tech in 2010, which are now, eleven years later, extremely outdated.

I felt on a mission to enlighten my fellow SLPs to the miracles of touch devices and the brand-new technology available. It was not just about my apps; it was about the fact that there was this incredible device that could give us access to therapy tools with the touch of a button. I became determined to integrate the mainstream iPhone and iPads into speech therapy sessions everywhere.

On April 3rd of 2010, shortly after my second and much better booth at the TSHA Convention, Apple announced the release of this brand-new device called the iPad. It was the very first iPad, and its arrival allowed my business to explode. I no longer had to convince my peers to use their personal iPhone for therapy. My job now was to teach them how to advocate so that their employer could purchase a device for them dedicated to therapy. They loved it, and I loved it that they loved it! A win all around for everyone.

As you have read, I had a lot happening at the same time. I am sure you do too. Things were happening fast for me, and I was hardly getting any sleep, but you know what? I felt great about getting things done. I was getting a taste of the high of taking charge of my entire day without a lot of restrictions and repetitive work that was hard for my personality type. I urge you to not wait until life is less overwhelming to start taking the small steps to build a life that comes from a place of joy; a life that is built around your strengths and all the things you have learned about yourself thus far.

Reflection Question: While you are busy being your amazing self, what are some things you would love to do, and what is the very first step that you need to take or that you can take this week to get there?

Chapter 12:

Finding Your Support System Elsewhere

"Technology is best when it brings people together."
Matt Mullenweg, Social Media Entrepreneur

As I write this book, I have to keep reminding myself that I am writing it with the ultimate goal to help you thrive as a minority SLP, despite all the barriers. In order to do that, I find myself thinking of every little detail that helped me get to where I am, regardless of whether or not it relates to being an immigrant, a Latina, or a minority. Yes, owning my own business was a shortcut for me, for sure. But having a support system was so important that you see it in the title of four chapters; this is one of them. I can never thank my support system enough. My girls know how much I appreciate them because I have made sure to honor them every time I can during the many conventions that our paths cross or by one of the many technological means we have at our disposal today. Unfortunately, the MSLP program only accepts a limited number of applicants a year, so we have to discuss other ways in which you can find your support network:

I want you to find your people too, and one of the options we have available these days is social media.

The beauty of social media, love it or hate it, is that it can help you connect with like-minded students and SLPs around the world. If you use your social media accounts for sharing your photos and connecting with friends, or even the eventual scrolling on Facebook, you may have a hard time envisioning how social media can help you build a support network. I am on the far end of the spectrum on this one. I met my husband online, so I am 100% biased to the power of the internet in bringing people together.

As the number of apps I published increased, so did my awareness of what I liked and what I could use some help with. Meanwhile, shortly after I created my GeekSLP Twitter account, I started engaging with a very small group of SLPs. That was the beginning of the #SLPeeps hashtag on Twitter. We connected, and as they were contributing to an SLP goal bank online, I offered to create an app in which they would be the authors and Smarty Ears would be the publisher. Five SLPs, which includes three who were internationally based, two in Canada and one in the Caribbean, became the first authors of Smarty Ears. The apps, called the SLP Goal Bank, gave birth to the concept that I would no longer create apps on my own.

"It was during this time as an SLPA student that I was introduced to the group of SLPs that have since become like family! The #SLPEEPS on Twitter. The OGs :) We still laugh together, cry together, celebrate together, write books together, and so much more! I will forever be grateful for this authentic community of humans." Ramya Kumar, Indian American SLP

What actually brings me joy in what I do is not the content building. It is the thought process of the innovation itself. I love coming up with creative technology to deliver speech and language content in an attractive and efficient way for you and the kids you support. That's where my talent and strength lies. From all that you know about me now, you know that the idea of sitting and writing 2,000 goals to be in a goal bank would completely drain my soul and likely be the cause of my death. Meanwhile, I also acknowledge my lack of competency in a variety of areas within our field; areas that I would love to create technology for, such as dysphagia and aphasia, just to name a couple. I have collaborated and published apps from at least fifteen authors that I met through social media.

Regardless of whether you connect via several of the groups on Facebook, Twitter, Instagram, or even ClubHouse, finding your people is a small but big part of your journey to not only thrive, but to share the joy that comes when you start killing it. Several of the stories you've already read or will read in this book came from connections I either made or reconnected on social media.

On Instagram, SLPs of color have been using the hashtags #slpsofcolor, #latinaslp or #bilingualSLPs when posting. That's another way to connect with SLPs who are starting to find their voice and use it to bring awareness, feel empowered, and empower the 14% of us in this field.

> "You just have to keep on looking for the person, the group, and your community. You have to build your community and be there for each other because there are so many things people go through, personally and professionally, and you just need that. You need somebody to sometimes just listen. You need someone there who's been through it." DM

While social media has not leveled the playing field completely, it has allowed for many of my talented colleagues to spread the word about their small businesses or side gigs and thrive in our field. I have plenty of stories about SLPs who started their businesses and are killing it without the money that big investors can pour into our field. They started small, harnessed social media, uncovered the power of online networking, collaborated with each other, and many are living fulfilling lives creating resources for our field.

Remember when I said that as a student, my point of support was the two minority professors in undergraduate (both not SLPs)? While in my graduate program, my support was also one of the bilingual clinical instructors. When I talked to the other voices in this book, this was a common occurrence for many of them. Obviously, this was not the case for everyone, and there are many exceptions to this; we are all humans after all. Finding minority faculty may be easier as an undergraduate since pretty much any other field has more diversity than ours. My gut advice says: open up and ask for support even outside of our field. Likely, they have been there too.

As a professional, I found myself doing exactly that. In my district, while there weren't any other bilingual SLPs on staff, there were plenty of other bilingual diagnosticians and special education secretaries. Since I quickly moved to an evaluator only position, those were my group of women. They helped me find my voice by proudly speaking Spanish with them as a group, and that was another powerful component in my healing journey.

There are a variety of ASHA Multicultural Constituents Groups (MCCGs) where you can find connections and meet new friends. Examples include the Asian Pacific Islander Speech-Language-Hearing Caucus, Haitian Caucus, Hispanic Caucus, L'GASP–GLBTQ Caucus, National Black Association for Speech-Language and Hearing (NBASLH), the Native American Caucus, and the South Asian Caucus. All these groups have Facebook pages which you can easily find in a Google search, and they hold meetings during the ASHA Convention. NBASLH has their own yearly conference too. You can visit their website to find future dates and locations. No, you don't have to be Black to attend!

> **"**In 2019, I went to the NBASLH mixer, and it was so nice to see SLPs of color being professionals and still having a good time. It was so refreshing seeing so many Black SLPs in a room." Leila Regio

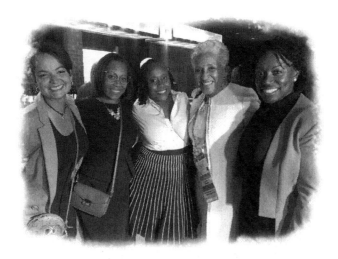

Finally, start putting yourself out there. This advice is for anyone, regardless of the demographics in your area. You could be in Tucker County, WV (the whitest county in America) or Aleutians West Census Area, Alaska (the most diverse county in America). You need to connect with SLPs at conferences in your state and other national conventions. Submit a presentation on the subject you are passionate about; heck, you could even present about your experience as an SLP and topics of diversity and biases in our profession. Walk the exhibit halls, and come visit me at my booth and chat! Start up a conversation with a colleague of color at these conferences, and don't be afraid to ask for their social media contact or start a connection. Too self-conscious? Yeah, it will take practice. Just last week I went to a concert alone because none of my friends liked either concerts or Latin concerts in particular. During the concert, I was lucky to sit next to a group of four girls. They were having a blast and included me. Two girls were from Bolivia and two were from Puerto Rico; by the end of the concert I asked for their contacts, and now I have a group of women who like concerts. I am an introvert, remember that? However, I have learned the power of finding like-minded people in many aspects of my life. It does not matter if it is someone to support us in times of struggle or to share and sing out loud during a music concert. Put yourself out there!

Reflection Question: Have you followed some of these tags on Instagram yet?

Barbara Fernandes

Chapter 13:

Finding Healing

"When you're different, sometimes you don't see the millions of people who accept you for what you are. All you notice is the person who doesn't." Jodi Picoult, *Change of Heart*

Muchachas, I am hitting my forties in a little over one year! Remember when you were younger and you naively looked up to people my age and thought that we had it all figured out? When I was twelve, I admired women who had a job, their own house, and a car. I was sure they had reached the peak of their lives.

Since I belong in the grown-up group now, I have realized that most grown-ups, like me, don't actually have things figured out. I am not referring to whether or not you have bought a house, earned degrees, have a car, and are debt free. I am talking about what is happening on the inside. I am talking about what is going on in your soul.

I am still surprised at how my emotions can sometimes catch me off guard when someone who was part of a toxic environment shows up again with their same behaviors much later in my life. You already read about a few of these moments, and I have even more to share.

My experiences hurt me, traumatized me, and scarred me. Recognizing these facts are important first steps, but you have to take several steps forward: You have to start doing the work to heal. I am still working on that. This book is a part of that healing journey that I didn't even know I was still on until two weeks ago.

> **"**I have lived meaningful stories as a speech-language pathologist, and these tales have brought me so much good. For now, in this season, I am honoring the ache, as well. The catalyst for this unearthing is not necessarily to be an informant for the underbelly of our profession. Rather, I am honoring certainties that I have inhaled for much too long, and it's making me sick. With this excavation, I can begin to reinvest in my sacred work with relentless authenticity and hope." Phuong Lien Palafox, Vietnamese Chinese American SLP

One of the most telling things about our need to heal, as I embarked on the journey to write this book, is the response I was getting as I asked others to share their own experiences and be vulnerable about their own journey. As I made my decision to write, I initially sent emails or texts to a close circle of SLPs who belong in the CLD group. Those texts led to other names of women I could speak with, and ultimately I ended up with a public invitation to anyone who wanted to share.

The responses I read from my email or texts sounded like:

"I am not sure I have the headspace to write about this right now because this is so triggering," or

"Real effing tears!"

Or Twitter replies like this:

Lou Rose 🎭 ⋯ she/they @petitetrout · 9m · · ·
Replying to @GeekBarbaraSLP
I'm very excited to read your book. I'm an ethnic and gender minority in grad school and actually had to quit my first externship due to racist, transphobic and ableist comments my supervisor kept making. It was a very hard situation mentally and emotionally

♡ 1   ↻   ♥ 1   ↑

As an educated empath, I know these words came from a place of trauma, pain, and struggle. I feel them. Before we can reduce the number of occurrences that require healing, we must acknowledge our own need to heal. As we help, we may forget that we need to help ourselves as well. Healing does not happen overnight. We heal a bit every time we speak up. Just as we become better clinicians at each ASHA Convention or training we attend, we become more healed versions of ourselves as we take steps toward it.

"As an undergraduate, I became an intern at a voice center. As someone who didn't yet know a lot about the limited number of minorities in this field, and as someone who grew up around diversity, it felt like a culture shock because there is not a lot of diversity in the spaces. This issue was incredibly evident in spaces for voice experts. I worked for eight hours a day there, doing unpaid labor as an intern just to increase my chances of getting accepted in a master's program. A variety of experiences constantly made me doubt my every move. I felt constantly pushed down and had my capacity questioned so often. I held on to these negative experiences for so long. I was so embarrassed. One of my friends, another Philippine undergraduate student, who was also an intern at this place, ended up quitting the field because of what we went through. It has been two years since I left the voice center, and I have been working to find healing. There are times that I still want to throw in the towel all from the scars that those two years left me with and come back to trigger me." Leila Regio

Leila's experiences didn't happen over ten years ago, it happened just two years ago. As I listened to her story, I ached knowing how she feels that it changed her; but I also cheer that she has found awareness and is working on speaking up and healing while still a student. For me, healing started the moment I had the courage to stand out and be unique, but that was just the start.

As my business was booming—my app library was growing to over thirty apps—I had many of my apps featured on Apple's New and Noteworthy chart, and at any given moment, I would have several apps in the top 100 Best- Selling educational apps on the App Store. I was quickly achieving the financial freedom of my dreams. Meanwhile, my video podcast and blog started to take on such a massive reach that I could not keep up with the many requests to be a paid speaker at state conventions, national and international conferences, and many professional development training sessions. I believe Barbara, as GeekSLP, the presenter, was born from the courage that I slowly gained through playing to my strengths by teaching SLPs about how to integrate technology in their practice through my video podcasts.

The struggle to put myself out there on video for the world to see was not without a lot of fear. On the business side, I had made a decision to hire native voiceover speakers to record the prompts for my apps, because I could not handle the likely rain of criticism that would follow from clinicians using an app with a foreign accented speech audio on it. Smarty Ears was receiving enough hate mail from SLPs simply for the fact that my accented voice, with the occasional incorrect preposition, was the voice on the video tutorials on the apps. I read every single one of those emails. They were hurtful. It took a lot of courage to put myself on video, sounding the way I do, for the same group of people who were sending me those messages.

On my GeekSLP Youtube channel, you can still find comments about my accent; however, what spoke louder to me was the fact that my channel grew to thousands of subscribers, and I was being invited to present. When I started my GeekSLP blog and podcast, my husband thought I was insane for taking on more work while I was so busy building and running my business. Looking back, I see that I was just doing what I know: advocating for the use of a technology that could transform our field. I also see that through putting myself out there, despite my several grammar mistakes and non-native accent, some people found value in what I had to say. Putting myself out there and becoming a public speaker was part of my healing. If I sat silently waiting for the xenophobic SLPs, who sat behind their keyboards, commenting on my videos, to be enlightened before starting anything, I would still be waiting. It is 2021, and we all have seen our fair share of cyberbullying.

I was at a much different place from the days in which I sat for hours with my accent reduction CDs, loathing myself in that process. I was at a much different place than when I agreed to have my speech evaluated, using the Goldman-Fristoe, at TCU during my first year as a graduate student.

Speaking and putting myself up to criticism was risky, but that's my MO. Healing has different processes for different people. Since my speech was a large contributor to having my soul crushed, it makes sense that being brave enough to put my voice out on video tutorials for my apps, creating a YouTube channel, or becoming a public speaker would be one of the stepping stones of my healing. This healing process may look different for you, depending on what you need healing from.

However, healing is not a one stop shop; it is a process. It starts with the awareness that you need healing in the first place or that you are still on that healing journey instead of pushing it all down, locking our pain in a chest of drawers, and throwing away the key.

We also need awareness of the impact of the words of others; both words that reached your ears a long time ago or words that will still come to face you in the present and can trigger your healing. Sometimes that awareness will take time to click in your brain and be recognized as "hmm… something was off here." You will read in future stories how often I had these experiences, but I was not yet in the mindspace to recognize them or to be aware of the impact they were having on me. I need you to get there sooner than I did.

I would like to say that when you have contributed, grown, or achieved a successful professional career, you will be immune to bullshit; unfortunately that has not been my experience. I am also aware that some of that bullshit isn't true bullshit; a lot of people still need to learn too. So I will classify some of that bullshit as cluelessness or ignorance. That's why I want you to be aware—so you can either acknowledge the bullshit or choose to make it a teachable moment. Let me tell you another story, so we can move from this theoretical debate into a more practical one.

During a recent virtual meeting with two employees, one new SLP employee and one who is not in our field, I had an experience that showed me that even healed parts of me may need a while to process the underlying message of a comment. At some point during the meeting, the conversation turned into a conversation about my accent, to which I commented that it was a long road for me to feel comfortable speaking up and using my own voice in business activities and resources. The white male SLP replied:

"That's crazy, Barb! Your accent is not even that bad."

I can't count the number of times I heard this from other SLPs. Qualifying an accent as good or bad, in and of itself, puts you in a position of having the ideal model of speech. People are qualifying the quality of an accent based on how closely it matches their own. Come on, sis, we are communication professionals; my accent is me, and you can't have the whole me without it. If you are a speaker of a more dominant version of English who is still trying to figure out what is wrong with qualifying accents according to the level in which they match the dominant dialect, think about how something similar could apply to you:

"Your [insert physical feature you can't live without] is not that bad!"

Our skin shades and physical features are neither better nor worse depending on how closely they match the dominant group; the same goes for accents. However, I did not realize this point until it was brought up a couple hours after the meeting by my other employee, who was also white and not an SLP. Despite this, he was obviously highly perceptive and much more aware of that conflict.

Was that a clueless moment for that male SLP or was it a xenophobic comment? I don't know, because I don't know him. However, could I not have used that moment as a teachable moment? Even if all I would have heard back would have been, "No! I didn't mean it that way," at least I would have let him know how he could have said it differently. I like giving people the benefit of the doubt but not to the extent of letting that benefit prevent helping them improve. He only worked for me for about four months. He was let go for reasons unrelated to this, so his departure meant I didn't have to dwell on the experience; but that also meant I never addressed how it made me feel. I didn't talk about it. I didn't process. I just added to the pile of hurt and kept moving forward. How much moving forward can we really do until our emotions catch up with us?

Healing is a journey, and all of us have a lot more to heal from than the things that happened in this field alone (especially if I open the umbrella to topics beyond the focus of this book, oh boy)! We are humans going through a full life beyond being a minority SLP; all those experiences add to our need to process, heal, and do a bit of self care. Psychotherapy, antidepressants, self-care, exercise, diet, writing, connection, standing up for others, reading

Sis, You Got This!

self-help books, calling friends and colleagues, listening to the experiences of the voices in this book, dancing, or becoming a role model all have their place in my healing; and I hope you have your own list of things to lead you to a more healed version of yourself each step of the way.

> **"**I have learned a lot of self-care. I am in a profession where I have to give caring advice, caring lessons, and I can't do that unless I take care of myself." DM

During my call with DM, she finished her one hour emotional chat with "Wow! This was great. I feel better for sharing all this with you. Thanks for listening, and I obviously should have been doing this more often."

Opening up and being able to share our hurt and pain can help us make sense of our painful experiences. This book is certainly doing that for me.

Regardless of how much healing I have done, some things still catch me off guard. However, being in a more aware state of mind leads me to the story about the final drop in the bucket. This drop led me to open Google Docs and type the outline of this book like a mad woman on the last day of the 2021 ASHA Convention.

Reflection Question: Can you think of something you are doing right now that is helping you find healing from something you have struggled with in the past? Maybe a hobby, time for yourself, therapy?

117

Barbara Fernandes

Chapter 14:

Sis, You Do Not Have to Change Your Answer

> "I not only have the right to stand up for myself, but I have the responsibility. I can't ask somebody else to stand up for me if I won't stand up for myself. And once you stand up for yourself, you'd be surprised that people say, 'Can I be of help?'"
> Maya Angelou

It may come to your surprise that the inspiration for this book came from two interactions on the first day of the 2021 ASHA Convention. In this chapter, I will share with you the final of the two interactions with a former faculty from one of the colleges I attended. The event that I am about to tell you about finally triggered the realization that no matter how much I had accomplished, there are moments in which the words of others still affect me and trigger unresolved conflicts within. This is why I led this section with awareness and healing. I didn't have either of those at the time of this event, at least not fully. However, this exchange brought about an awareness of an area that needed my healing chain reaction. This book is it. I hope this book also inspires you to find your own healing reaction, hopefully much sooner than mine.

On a cold Friday night in Washington, DC, I was celebrating life with my closest circle from the Minority Student Leadership Program at an event honoring Dr. Tommie Robinson Jr. It was held at the bar at the Marriott hotel connected to the convention center.

These events usually take place on Thursday or Friday evenings during every ASHA convention; this is also when all the different multicultural constituent groups have their open houses. There is also an event called MC2 which is an evening event for all the multicultural constituent groups. The rooms in which these events take place have a different vibe. The NBASLH open house has always been a place of belonging for me. They always feel very different from the rest of the convention. There, I was not part of the "minority group;" it was a room filled with our people—people who can feel me even if they don't know me. The 8.5% in our field account for the 95% in that room. My people are my fellow MSLP alum, my culturally, ethnically and linguistically diverse friends, and our allies. These evening events during the ASHA Convention, besides being the most fun, have always been the safest place for me to be every single year. If you ever get a chance to attend an ASHA Convention, keep an eye out for these Friday evening events.

I was sitting at the bar, enjoying a glass of wine and chatting with lifelong friends, overlooking this wonderful celebration. When I turned to my left, I saw a former professor of mine. She had a smile on her face, and after the first few minutes of small talk, she asked:

"Do you miss your time at TCU?"

To which I promptly answered, "I do not."

Unhappy with my answer, and without any hesitancy, she made an interesting request:

"Let's try that again, but this time more diplomatically."

I want to insert the shocked emoji face. Just go ahead and imagine it. Remember a few moments earlier when I talked about how sometimes I give people the grace that their comments are a result of cluelessness? At first, this was one of those moments. I stood my ground and attempted to explain to her that my experience was not overall positive, despite the excellent academic education I received. I proceeded and asked, "Do you also ask this of other students?"

Her response alluded to the fact that while other students may not miss the academic requirements, they miss the camaraderie. To which I replied:

"Well, that was not my experience. I was always left out when materials and resources were being shared between the students, including materials and answers for your exams. The same applies to study groups and the everyday life that my white peers were able to share among themselves."

To which she asked, "And whose fault is that?" with a tone that took me several moments to process before she was called away by someone else to greet her.

As I stood there, somewhat in shock, all sorts of emotions filled up my body. I realized that I was experiencing one of those moments in which the room was empty, and there were just the two of us in there. As she walked away, I slowly came back to realizing we were in a room with hundreds of people. Two women, who I didn't yet know, approached me and said:

"We saw the whole thing. Good for you for standing up. I could not believe how inappropriate that was."

Those two women, who have become a part of my life, caught me off guard, and without realizing it, they disarmed me. Thank you for seeing me, Samantha Ghali and Teresa Girolamo. The tears started to roll down my face. I turned around, so nobody else would see me crying. I took a couple minutes to compose myself and brush that interaction off (at least externally). At that moment, I thought of all the times that I tried, all the times I extended a hand, all the times I attempted. This moment crashed on my face saying: None of it mattered.

In moments of trauma, reality can get cloudy. Our minds are designed to shut down and forget hurtful words, so we can keep moving. That's why witness accounts have so much power:

> "The room was packed, and I was first facing the bar, where I saw you sitting having a drink, minding your own business. A person squeezed by, and I saw her begin to talk to you. I eventually had to pivot away from the bar due to the comings and goings of the room, but could still hear both of your voices (you were less than two feet away from me). I was being introduced to someone new, but I heard her voice rising

in volume—you never raised your voice once. I couldn't hear much, but I could tell there was some kind of disagreement going on. I could also tell that the discussion was between a white person and a person who is a minority.

I kept having to tune in and out of each conversation, because I couldn't immediately excuse myself, but I knew I still had to keep an ear out for what was going on behind me. She said some inappropriate things that made me turn around and feel like something was not right about the interaction.

Despite her impropriety, you still showed her respect and deference. You did not argue back, but acquiesced to her words. That's when I knew I had to wrap up my conversation immediately, and I informed the colleague standing next to me that we had best go over to check on the person (you) because what had just gone down was not okay."

As much as I felt alone at that moment, I am grateful that the room was packed. One witness is good, two is even better . . .

"As a third-party observer to that interaction, the exchange shook me to my core (and I say this as a spouse to an active duty military officer who assisted with the humanitarian evacuation out of Afghanistan). Just about every minority in CSD I know has had the distinct displeasure of having others from the dominant majority attempt to silence them. Speaking truth to power is an essential act of survival, and when others try to deny truths which cannot possibly belong to them, they are, in effect, trying to strip minorities of their dignity. Such acts do not align to the values central to speech-language-hearing, or more broadly, to the values that motivate many—like my spouse—to serve their country." Teresa Girolamo, PhD

There is a lot to unpack from that five minute exchange. Let me try to do that, one thing at a time. As I was in the middle of experiencing that moment, the first word that came to my mind was "gaslighting." As you know by now, I have recently become an avid reader of personality tests and psychological profiles. When it comes to human interactions, gaslighting is one of the words that it took me a while to understand. When someone gaslights you, they want to rewrite your experience and negate your feelings as invalid by attempting to create a distorted version of your own reality. Gaslighting may look like phrases such as *You are being sensitive* or *It was not that bad, you are overreacting*, among others.

Our experiences of racism, biases, isolation, and microaggressions are real. It took me fifteen years to speak up and stand up about my experiences. Nobody will silence me now. I don't want you to wait fifteen years to start telling your truth and sharing your experiences. We are free to talk about them, even if institutions won't look good in that process. If they wanted to look good, they should have done better. We all can share the aspiration that, while institutions may have failed us, there is hope for the future; but they can't keep the lid on the past. When we are forced to change our reality, that's when we must be able to stand our ground and speak our truth.

I have come to be okay and accept the times people have called me "too sensitive." I am not sure when labeling someone as sensitive became an attempt at pointing out a flaw because I love being sensitive to my own needs and the needs of others around me. That's not a bad thing. That's a great thing! I am an empath, and I can pick up on people's energy like it is no one's business. I have learned to use my sensitivity to navigate the world and walk away from things not meant for me. That's a brand-new skill though.

When it comes to my "undiplomatic answer," she is right if being diplomatic is only achieved by giving the answer she wanted to hear. My gut instinct is to say, "I am not interested in cultivating 'diplomacy,' especially if it requires me to rewrite my own experiences."

The reality is that I was in fact being diplomatic. As I sat there being challenged about my experience, it took a lot of effort and energy to find the correct words to get my message across. It takes a huge mental effort to respond in a way that could have the most impact—especially when emotions run high. But you know what? I handled it. I had all the reasons to have lost it, but I didn't.

Real diplomacy doesn't come from an exchange of fakeries. Diplomacy should mean that people are brought to the table to be honest and reflective and work towards a common good. It shouldn't smell like it lives off of "quid pro quos." If a university and its individual faculty have any desire to do better, they should recognize and acknowledge its alumni's scars without needing consolation from receiving criticism. Whether dealing with a university or a person, it's not a healthy relationship when you have to console the aggressor.

Every university should be genuinely interested in the experiences of its alumni, both during and after graduation, to ensure that they are delivering the best experience possible. How can they improve if they want to be outright dismissive of negative experiences? I was there at the table for that common good. I wasn't particularly in the mood, but I was still there because I know universities need to be thinking more about this. Metaphorically, no one joined me at that table for the greater good. I couldn't be diplomatic because my truth was treated as unworthy of being listened to.

It is a strange thing when people think the burden of diplomacy should rest completely on the shoulders of the one with less power. It's even stranger when the side with the most power doesn't act like it needs to have the interest of showing up and listening. Do we not see how much strength it even takes to speak up against a large organization? Was there ever a genuine curiosity to hear whatever answer I gave? Who was actually being undiplomatic in that exchange?

I avoid confrontation like the plague. It's just not my MO. I avoid it so much that I have lost business dealings because I knew that one confrontational incident would ruin my ability to deal with a lot of other business things. I hired someone to handle all the direct confrontation I would have to deal with in my business. So, when I tell you that I had chosen to gracefully acknowledge and have casual encounters with everyone who has put me down up to this point, please believe me. Most of me would prefer to not engage in any type of confrontation, but she came into my space. In fact, one of the safest and most special places for me for sixteen years was any given ASHA Convention.

However, there is a big difference between the tranquil energy of a graceful hello when you see these people later in life and under different circumstances, as they swing by your booth or cross paths with you at a convention, and the necessary response you have to their questions when they ask you to change your answer about how you experienced life with them in your past. Sister, give any darn answer you feel like; you do not need to change your answer. You do not need to change your responses to make institutions look better, no matter how much better they are doing now. Your experiences were real, and they are all yours.

> "When I started my master's program, I was twenty-nine years old and I had seven years of experience as a classroom teacher. I was confident about all the life experiences I had under my belt that could help me stand out among the young and inexperienced first year graduate students. By the end of the program, I was taking antidepressants." DM, Black SLP from NY

By the end of my graduate program, I was on antidepressants too. In my humble opinion, depression should not come with those two letters after your name when you've earned a degree.

The fact that I am grateful for all I have learned, the numerous positive experiences I had, and the impact that others within the institutions that helped me achieve my goals had on me does not change the scars it left me with. Yes, my experiences during my graduate program were an upgrade from my undergraduate experiences, but they still had a severely negative impact on me. Looking back, I wish I had asked what she meant by, "And whose fault is that?" I wasn't sure if she was referring to the fact that it was my fault or the other students' fault. If it was the first, which is how I interpreted it at the time, then shame on her. If it was the latter, then as a business owner, I say: The culture is always determined by leadership.

At some point in that exchange, my ex-professor and now colleague (a point that she might have forgotten) stated that the university is doing so much better since I left and that I needed to give them credit for it. I could feel the undertone that it came with. It is the same undertone that I have discussed before: the one they use when they want to make you feel like you owe them something for the fact that they finally started doing what is right. We don't owe them a pat on their backs!

There is an underlying assumption here that institutions doing the bare minimum to provide decent culturally-sensitive education or infusing the token diverse staff are things that we need to give them credit for, as if they were doing us a favor. They are not doing us a favor—that is the bare minimum. All of this feels really reminiscent of my experience as a mother of children who receive special education services. I am not asking for favors when my kids receive the accommodations or special services they need in order to learn and thrive.

Diversity produces a completely different culture within institutions that should be valued and honored for what it is. Diversity enriches institutional culture and strengthens any community. They are not doing us any favors. We do not need to praise the least racist person in the room because they are not chaining anyone to the table anymore.

Yes, I am happy to hear that the institution I received my master's degree from might be doing better in this aspect; however, that does not change my feeling that as an institution geared towards providing an inclusive educational experience, they have never been interested in engaging with me about my experience, despite attempts from my end.

That colleague and I never got a chance to finish the conversation that night in the way I would have liked to in order to attempt to make a meaningful impact for the future. I needed time to process that experience anyway. It was important to me to not feel like I left things unsaid. I am an advocate; I want the future students to have more support and a sense of belonging.

The morning after that interaction, I sent that faculty member an email, saying that I would love to continue that conversation. I invited her to meet during the ASHA Convention by telling her that she could find me at my booth or that I would happily meet her elsewhere. Unfortunately, we never had closure because she didn't respond to the email until I was back. She vaguely stated that we may resume the conversation in the future; but she clearly isn't interested in doing so. Even though I believe she should have been more interested by being the one to reach out to make the program better for future students, I was the one who took it upon myself to make myself available to her. I still live in the same area, so we didn't even have to talk at ASHA. I want to give grace and the opportunity to colleges to ask themselves the question, "How can we do better? How can we make sure that our current students don't answer the same way you did?" instead of asking alumni to pretend their experiences weren't real.

Did I consider dedicating this book to her? Yeah, some of you even suggested I do that. But in the end, this book is dedicated to us who have kept swimming and to the ones who drowned, like the bilingual Latina SLP-A who was my assistant in my public school position; she drowned during her time as a graduate student at TCU and never finished her degree. She, like all of us, deserved more support to be the SLP we once dreamed we could become.

This entire chapter represents a lot. It contributed to inspiring me to write a book. It opened my eyes about the fact that I am still not seen as an equal colleague. It reminded me that sometimes you need people around to support you no matter how high you have climbed, and it reminded me that no matter how high we climb, some people will never recognize it. Speaking of recognition . . .

Reflection Question: Have you thought about how you would respond when a faculty asks you about your experience?

Barbara Fernandes

Chapter 15:

Is the 91.5% Only Recognizing Their Own?

"If you elect to join the herd you are immune. To be accepted and appreciated you must nullify yourself, make yourself indistinguishable from the herd. You may dream, if you dream alike." Henry Miller, *Tropic of Capricorn*

The goal of this book is not to create an "us versus them" mentality at all, which is why I asked all of us to recognize our own biases in the previous chapters. We all could use more recognition of our own biases and stereotypes toward different racial and ethnic groups. However, I can't shake the feeling that minority speech-language pathologists are still getting the short end of the stick, especially when it comes to recognition for our accomplishments. We obviously don't do the work we do for recognition, but I know seeing our faces in awards is another way in which we can show the younger versions of ourselves what we are bringing to the table.

You may remember that a few years ago, in 2015, the hashtag trending was #OscarsSoWhite given the fact that the industry was failing to celebrate a diversity that already somewhat existed. All twenty actor nominees were white in 2015. The year after that Twitter hashtag trended, an entire industry recognized the need to invest in high-budget films that promoted diversity.

The result: *Black Panther*, *Coco*, and *Get Out*, just to name a few. While that crisis is resting for the time being, a new crisis is taking over the industry, and this new crisis, that I just stumbled upon while writing this book, has everything to do with the point I am trying to make in this chapter.

The latest Golden Globe™ controversy is about the lack of diversity among the deciding members, and it makes total sense. In 2021, out of the eighty-four members of the Associated Press that made the decision, not a single one is Black. Why would it be important to have diversity among the people who are selecting the award recipients? I believe it's because we need to recognize the implicit bias we all may have when making decisions about who we are recognizing and the value that their contributions bring.

When it comes to recognition within our field, I wonder how much we are mirroring what happened and what is still happening in mainstream media. It seems obvious to me that if in a group of ten people, nine of them are white, either as the ones in a nominating role or decision-making role, and given all the biases, women of color will end up not being recognized. Are we in a cycle of suffering from the internal bias of the 91.5% making decisions about who is worthy of recognition in this field? In that racial and ethnic decision making, are we showing young clinicians and students of color that we SEE them too?

Am I alone in this feeling of being invisible?

A lot of progress and initiative at the national level has been made to reduce this bias. When it comes to our professional association, I have seen more and more diverse faces during the award ceremonies at the ASHA Conventions in the last few years, and that's a reason to celebrate. As I looked at the ASHA Convention awardees history, it was empowering to see the gradual shift of shades from white to brown as the years progressed. Go ahead and do it yourself too; it is readily available on their website. As someone who has attended the ASHA Convention nearly every single year since 2005, I can see and feel the difference in the posters and materials advertising award winners over the years. We have clearly made enough noise at the national level to spark some change, and people are listening. But most importantly, we had amazing people within the non-White group who took it upon themselves to run for offices and contribute to making the change happen.

The problem came in when I started to look at this issue at the state level and within universities. Looking at this data for every state is a massive task. I will leave it for one of you to go after as your student thesis in your education journey.

In order to at least attempt to look for some of the information regarding nominations and awards demographics within our field, I focused on looking at the websites for associations for the big diverse states like Texas, California, New York, or Florida. I could not find any record of their diversity count for past nominations, awardees, or decision makers for the awards on any of their websites. California's website listed the names of the nomination board committee but not the procedures. Texas listed the procedures but not the names of deciding members. Florida didn't list either.

The bottom line is that none of the states had the pertinent information available on their website in order to determine if there is a bias. Before we can even discuss a potential bias problem, I can tell you that we at least have a problem with transparency. In fact, the issue of transparency is one that has caused a lot of controversy in our field, especially when it comes to how decisions are made and how things work at the professional level of our state and national associations.

As this data is not easily found, and this is not a research article, we will continue with our anecdotal accounts. This data issue indicates a need for a couple things: people asking questions and making some noise at the different state associations and more transparency of this information. Even for our national association, which is doing an outstanding job in this aspect, I still want to know some things, and I want these things updated yearly on their website: Who is making these decisions, what are the demographics of the people making these decisions, what are the demographics of the nominees, and what are the demographics of the award recipients? Having transparency is a start.

Between me and my businesses, I have received my fair share of awards. However, none of my recognitions have come from our field or from any of the colleges I attended. TCU reached out to me to write a story about me and my entrepreneurial success for the TCU Magazine; but again, that recognition did not come from the CSD department within TCU. Racism and bias are everywhere, but why has it rarely impacted my ability to be recognized outside of our field as much as it does within our field? It feels as if our field is slow in catching up with the world.

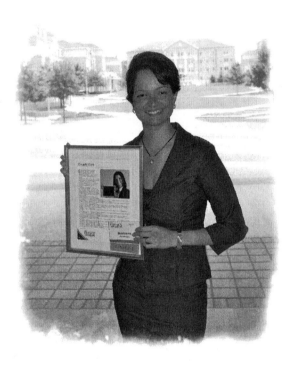

Around 2011, I had the pleasure of receiving an award at TCU for being a finalist in the Impact Awards. But, girl, don't get your hopes up; that was just the venue. It had nothing to do with the CSD department or TCU. I made a point to walk next door to the CSD clinic to visit, show them my award and visit with the administrative staff. Over the years, Smarty Ears, as a business, has received a variety of awards—but not Barbara Fernandes, who was the person behind all those creations. I promise, guys, that this is not about my ego talking; I already had a one on one with it to make sure.

Now, you might be wondering: Are universities or state organizations recognizing anyone? Yes! In this process, I reached out to the two universities I attended to see if recognizing alums was even a thing, and if so, whether or not they have demographic information on who received these nominations. TCU confirmed that "the department has a long history of internal and external recognition of our faculty, students, and alumni."

Temple University has nominated several CSD alumni for awards, but none of them have received an award from the college yet. When I asked about the demographics of nominees, I was told that the data was difficult to find, or I got no response at all. Giving the benefit of the doubt, it is possible that the data really was hard to find instead of scary to share, especially after I told why I needed it. But we don't know because these decisions are made behind closed doors by a faculty that is primarily not diverse.

One white SLP created two apps, both of which are versions of two apps I had created myself three years prior, and she was recognized by the Utah Association for her outstanding clinical achievement in 2014. By that year, I had not only created the original versions of those two apps that she was awarded for, but I had actually published over thirty apps and an entire symbol set library—Smarty Symbols.

Am I really that invisible?

This is not about discrediting anyone's awards or recognitions for their contributions to the field. It's about bringing up the question of whether people with a diverse background are being properly recognized for their contribution to this field; and if not, whether it is an issue of representation among the decision makers or a matter of the person needing not only to achieve a lot more than our white counterparts, but also to belong in the decision makers's group in order to be recognized. We need a seat at the table.

In the last chapter, I shared about my alleged lack of diplomacy in my answer to a faculty member, and I started to wonder how that statement might be related to this issue of recognition. We all have a bias toward recognizing those who belong to our group. Here, people of color, especially the ones who never belonged and who struggled and decided to either isolate themselves or speak up, will face yet another barrier towards the recognition of our contributions. As if the 91.5% judging bias weren't enough, we must stay quiet, put on a smile, and conform to their expectations if we want to be seen and recognized. We must keep the lid down on our experiences and go about them quietly.

As we voice our struggles or start conversations for change and stop conforming, are their perceptions of us as undiplomatic having this much impact? Do I need to conform just so I can belong and be recognized? I shouldn't have to. And if the people making these decisions see me as an outsider, did I ever stand a chance regardless of my intention to conform? As Brené Brown would say, "True belonging is being able to be who you are and still be accepted as one of them." This may be one of the reasons why feeling the lack of belonging has sat with me for fifteen years since I received my last degree.

For the past several years, at the Texas Speech and Hearing Association Convention (TSHA), universities have held their open house events for faculty, current students, and alumni. As you might expect, as someone who never quite felt like one of their own, those were not events I was ever eager to attend. Many years ago, probably within two to three years of my graduation, one of my peers invited me to attend one of these receptions with her. I was so out of place, you guys! It was worse than my college days. We all know the feeling of people being cordial but not seeing you as one of their own. That's exactly how I felt in that space. I have attended every single TSHA Convention since, and I have yet to ever return to one of those open house events.

Even more recently, I made a business decision to donate all Smarty Ears apps to colleges around the USA. Our team has donated hundreds of thousands of dollars worth of apps to hundreds of colleges. It is a tedious process on both ends. However, colleges are always very grateful and appreciative of our gesture. Which college was the only one to let this process fail? Yeah, the one I went to. The one I had a personal relationship with.

My feelings of lack of appreciation and belonging didn't leave when I graduated. Every attempt I made to reach out, even though I strongly believe that the majority group should be responsible for that process, has failed.

I am guilty of not dedicating more time to networking and campaigning. For some, this is what diplomacy looks like: a campaign. You must give yourself an agreeable image for those who hold the power to judge your worthiness to let you in the inner circle. It is like judging an author based off of her personal charisma for her worthiness to win the Nobel Prize in Literature, instead of *gasp* actually reading her work. Maybe every award-giving body functions like that to some extent, but that would explain why so many organizations are leaving out talent. I haven't had an interest in an active campaign of networking. I've been the personality that, with each passing year, is looking for more genuine connections. I seek genuine connections, not only in my personal life, but also in business. If diplomacy means that I need to act like a political candidate, making myself overly agreeable and not showing up as my genuine self—were any of these "diplomatic" relations worth the price for simply being given a chance to be treated fairly? Is attending these events in which I was made to feel uncomfortable as an outsider worth the possible benefits? Not for me.

I am a world traveler and an immigrant who struggles with belonging in a weird way; I belong nowhere and everywhere. I feel like an insider anywhere on this planet. As a citizen of the world, the bar for people making me feel like I don't belong is very high. I have yet to feel welcomed or feel that type of college pride my TCU fellows in other fields experience.

There is a lot of room for us to navigate in between giving the answer that makes colleges or places of work look good and setting up posters and gathering a group to protest in front of their place of business demanding change. There are many ways that we can assert our truths while maintaining an open channel of communication that leads to growth and change in this field. None of these actions should impact or weigh on their ability to recognize our contributions, even if I did set up a protest tent in front of their clinic, but they do. This fear of retaliation is the reason one of my colleagues who contributed to my book asked to contribute anonymously. My book is a safe place for sharing however we wish, and while I did not have a problem with them contributing this way, the simple fact that we fear retaliation for speaking our truth and sharing our stories is reason for alarm in my opinion.

Did you feel a little bit of resentment from me as you read this chapter? Maybe. Over sixty apps later, still no recognition from my colleges, state association, national association, or anywhere within this field really. All my recognition comes from the technology industry. However, the resentment is not toward the other people receiving the awards; it is, with a newfound awareness, toward the systemic handicap that women coming from diverse backgrounds are facing. This handicap occurs either because the men or white women are both the decision makers and award winners within our field, because of the apparent bias in nominations toward people within our group, or because we burned bridges speaking up or walking away from places we weren't welcomed.

Another hypothesis for what could be contributing to the lack of recognition among POC is that minority professionals are not engaging in the nomination procedures as much as our white counterparts. If so, come on, sister, get working. Just kidding. I do have one piece of anecdotal evidence to the contrary. A few years ago, Mai Ling Chan, submitted a nomination for me to be considered for an ASHA award. I am not sure what exactly it was or what it encompassed. She did all the groundwork that apparently is involved in this. While it has been several years since, and ASHA has been doing much better, there is still a lot that we don't know. Unless we get data on demographics of the nominees, we will never know the data points between percentage nominated versus the percentage awarded to answer this hypothesis. If anyone else here is looking for yet another research idea, you're welcome.

This leads me to the most important point in this chapter: the need for awareness, transparency, and unity—all of which, in my opinion, appear to be essential in the process of improving our prospects in our field. Unity can be achieved by recognizing the incredible amount of disheartening experiences we have shared, regardless of our individual differences. This is about finding common ground.

There is one aspect in which we can also find common ground with white women in this field: men are still leading this field and receiving most of our awards. That's our conversation for the next chapter.

Reflection Question: Can you think of an SLP of color who you would like to honor?

Chapter 16:

Can We Also Talk about the Male Role in Our Field?

"We need to stop buying into the myth about gender equality. It isn't a reality yet. Today, women make up half of the US workforce, but the average working woman earns only 77 percent of what the average working man makes. But unless women and men both say this is unacceptable, things will not change." Beyonce Knowles

Since we are discussing recognition bias in our field, I wanted to share another rabbit hole that I found myself dwelling on and frustrated about as I embarked on this book writing journey: the role of men in our field. You would think that in a profession in which women are the overwhelming majority, being a female SLP may make you feel grateful to be in the majority group (at least when it comes to your gender), right? We can be a minority in terms of our ethnicity or race but in the majority when it comes to gender, right? Not so fast! Even though speech-language pathology is ranked the third profession with the least number of men, only behind preschool teachers and dental hygienists, men are leading this field everywhere.

I am not an anthropologist, but I can't shake the feeling, especially as a businesswoman in this field, that being a female SLP does not necessarily make me feel warm and fuzzy inside or empowered. Should we start considering being a woman as another facet of being a minority in this field? In my humble opinion, absolutely! Sexism in this field is real. That's why I am constantly dealing with the 4% always in a position of power. The men are making decisions in academia as chairs of departments, starting and running businesses in our field, receiving recognition, and taking on positions of prestige within the associations in numbers completely disproportionate to their representation—not to mention the non-SLP men who come as investors in our field as well.

I understand that this is probably the most controversial part of this book, especially because we do need more men to support young students with their communication needs. One of ASHA's strategic objectives is to increase the percentage of men in this field (ASHA, 2021). While it is a worthy and needed objective, it needs to be reached with an awareness of the trends that will continue to keep women underrepresented in positions of power. The two goals are not conflicting. We can recruit more men as clinicians, while keeping an eye on our own bias toward only bringing them to lead the field. When the time comes that men are no longer grossly overrepresented in awards, decision-making positions, or positions of power despite the minuscule piece of the pie that they represent in this field, then this no longer becomes a topic worthy of discussion. Until then, we have to address this elephant in the room that I, somehow, could not find a mention of anywhere in my limited research.

In order to try to validate my feelings of contrast in this area when comparing the numeric minority of women of color and the numeric minority of men in this field, I want to look at the definition of being a minority. The definition that came closer to explaining and justifying my feelings were from Britannica: "minority, a culturally, ethnically, or racially distinct group that coexists with but is subordinate to a more dominant group. As such, minority status does not necessarily correlate to population. In some cases one or more so-called minority groups may have a population many times the size of the dominating group, as was the case in South Africa under apartheid." https://www.britannica.com/topic/minority That's not just a "South Africa during the apartheid" issue; this is a current issue within our field. As far as I can feel, we can be the majority gender and still be "minoritized" in our role as females in this field.

How is it that in a profession that is 4.7% male, we often see them in many decision-making positions, as if they are playing a bigger role in the shape of this profession in comparison to the 95.3% of the women?

Let's look at some shocking statistics to make this even more evident. Even thinking about the 2021 ASHA's Honors Awardees of the association (ASHA, 2021), in a profession that is 4.7% male; seven out of eleven awardees were male! From 1976 to 2021, we had fourteen male (31% over 44 years) ASHA presidents. Things have gotten a lot better since 2011, with the last ten ASHA presidents being female. In eleven years of the Clinical Aphasiology Conference, only eleven out of thirty-seven awardees were female. In eleven years of the Academy of Aphasia, five out of eleven were female (65% were male).

How does this translate to our individual reality as we navigate this field? As I graduated from my undergraduate, the new chair was a male; during my master's program, the chair was a male; and the upcoming chair was also a man. Would you like to guess the gender of the current chair at that university? Yes, he is a man too. There was a one in twenty chance that the person replacing a male chair would be a man, but he was and is again! I wondered, what is the chance of having three one-in-twenty chances in a row? So I asked Twitter, and here is the answer:

Matthew Winn @matt_with_ears · Dec 8 ···
Replying to @GeekBarbaraSLP and @CherylStephens
It would be 0.0025%, given your numbers. 25 times out of a million. That is wild.

Prior to me bringing my first child into this world, my husband would attend every convention with me, both our national convention as well as the many state conventions in which we decided to exhibit. One of the most irritating things that happened during these conventions were other men, SLPs or not, coming to my booth to attempt to do business and directing all their conversation toward my husband. It didn't matter how often my husband would openly say, "She is the boss. I am just the helper," the conversations were still directed at him.

Don't get me wrong, my husband has been my sidekick since 2008. He is my biggest supporter, and I could write an entire chapter just about the importance of finding a partner that honestly supports your growth, healing, and success. He has cared for our kids as I traveled for work, as I stayed up working on my next business project, or as I sat in the office writing this book. However this is not a book about my relationship advice. Maybe I will write that one later in life.

My husband, Jonathan, who is an English teacher by trade, has created content for a couple of Smarty Ears apps as well. He has worked full time on Smarty Ears since 2011 when our business started to explode. He is a part of my business, but this is my business. I hire, fire, manage, and I am the final decision maker. However, as a business woman in a white majority and clearly male-driven field, the vast majority of company meetings for partnerships are with men, who often try to exert their control over me. Several comments I have heard over the years have been sexist, patronizing, or outright offensive.

It is frustrating. The fact that I have gotten used to it or that I have had my husband join in many meetings just as a male figure on my side of the table is alarming. Let me remind you: I am in a field that is 96% female, and I am not doing much business outside of our field.

One year at a TSHA Convention, I was at my booth when the chair of a CSD department, a man, stopped by to chat. At the time, I had just found a new groove: applying for research and development grants. Many of these grants require a higher institution sub-contractor who will often do the research portion of your new technology development. I had sent in three applications, and since he was the chair of a Dallas/Fort Worth institution, I told him that I was applying and was looking for university partners. His response:

"Have you actually gotten a grant yet? They are very hard to get."

I can somewhat remember him saying that he had attempted it himself, but I could be also totally making this last part up. However, what I clearly remember was the undertone. A tone of complete lack of confidence that I (make it an emphatic *I* as you read this) could ever get a grant like that. As an empath, I could feel the undertone with every fiber of my body. Since he was a man, I am not sure if the undertone of a complete lack of faith and interest in having anyone at the university involved was a tone directed toward me as a woman or me as a minority woman.

We often think of sexism, gender or racial bias, or discrimination as a blatant vocal demonstration. Those still happen too. However, I have come to realize that the undertone we feel when we are subtly questioned about our ability to achieve is just as impactful. I have found this type of subtle remark, often built-in on the tone, one of the hardest to identify. At times, I found myself taking a few moments and sitting with and processing that feeling of *what just happened?* to come to the conclusion. Sometimes I walk away from conversations with that feeling in my stomach, will drive home wondering what was wrong, and then it'll hit me: "Ah! It was the tone and the vibe. He really didn't think I could pull it off, did he? He didn't think I could receive that grant since he could not have done it himself."

This subtle message will get under your skin and destroy you and your self-esteem, all without you even noticing it just happened. That's the same undertone I heard from the faculty at the ASHA Convention. If any profession could understand the difference between vocabulary and tone while using the same vocabulary, you are in the profession that absolutely knows that difference. The worst part is that you can't say there was anything wrong with the words used in order to fight back or write that email questioning. All you have is a feeling, and that often has no leg to stand on.

Don't worry, I did get that grant from the National Institute of Health just two months after this exchange. Wink.

We may not think that having men as owners or CEOs of the businesses SLPs buy things from has any impact on us or how we do business or deliver therapy; but as a business owner myself, I can tell you that it is absolutely impactful. Leaders of businesses are ultimately deciding which ideas get funded, what gets represented in the products you consume, which books get published, which articles get written about, what goes on their blog section, and all the way down to what or who is or isn't included in visual support. It impacts every single aspect of the materials you buy. Yes, support our female-owned or women-led businesses.

Remember when I heard, "Would you rather be the sole owner of an x million dollar company or the owner of a 10x million dollar company with partners?" The person who asked me this is a man. His business decisions are different from mine as a woman with different priorities and different points of view. I could tell that he could not grasp how I could pick the option with the least financial reward but the freedom to drive my business in the direction I find most appropriate. However, don't let my decision to pick the option with the least financial return fool you. "Private technology companies led by women are more capital-efficient, achieving 35% higher return on investment" (Forbes.com).

We have covered topics from male SLPs receiving awards to leading university departments to male-led SLP businesses. If we combine the fact that this is one of the whitest fields with the facts that men are absolutely driving this field, I can't help but come to the conclusion that this is a white male driven field! This sentence by itself is insane. Men leading a field that has roughly 88.4% white women has to mean that the women are the ones putting the men in a position of power, control, and status. In this case the implicit gender bias is working against the numeric majority, making it impossible for a minority female to fulfill this role.

Remember how I have asked you to look at the common ground? This time, I am shining a light on the common ground women in our field have, regardless of their racial and ethnic background. Finding common ground is powerful in bringing people together. We have many changes to bring about, and this is one where we can get the 91.5% to empathize rather than sympathize.

As I close this chapter, I want to raise a glass to all the women who are kicking butt in this field by starting businesses, running them, hiring women for leadership positions, writing articles, editing research articles, chairing CSD programs, applying for funding and receiving it, becoming ASHA CEOs or presidents, and achieving many other leadership roles in our field; and I will raise two for you minority women who are doing all of that too, despite the many barriers, words of oppression, and systemic disadvantages you have faced so far.

P.S. It is okay if you cried reading this last paragraph. I sobbed while writing it.

Reflection Question: Is it time for us to start advocating for ASHA and state associations to start grants for women to get a head start on their businesses?

Chapter 17:

SLP Business Ownership and Innovation

"Don't let anyone rob you of your imagination, your creativity, or your curiosity. It's your place in the world; it's your life. Go on and do all you can with it, and make it the life you want to live."
Mae Jemison, First Black Astronaut

Amiga, I want to see you thrive. Now that I have pushed you to think about what makes you unique in this field and have shared about the barriers we still face, it is time to share the juicy stuff that helped me thrive and live the professional life of my dreams. It was a road filled with mistakes and lessons, but it provided a lot of growth. I hope this will inspire you to join me in the pursuit of discovering what drives you and then following that journey. Maybe you'll get inspired to become the chair of a CSD program department, the next president of ASHA or of your state association, become the lead SLP in your district, or pursue any other leadership roles that you might have discovered along the way. Who knows, maybe you will feel inspired to start your own SLP business or create a new innovative product. If you ever do, please write to me and share whatever glass ceiling you might be breaking; I want to raise a glass for you when you find what moves you and discover the success it will bring.

I am not sure if it is my neurodiversity, my personality type, my background, or my mistakes and lessons, but one of my favorite things about my job is when I am in the groove phase of a new project. Some days, I wake up at five o'clock in the morning to work, get my kids ready for school, and continue to work fifteen hours straight until it is time to watch a movie to wind down and pass out. I love the adrenaline of a new challenge and the daily changes that owning two businesses in this field brings. I find myself swallowing my food faster (dysphagia peeps, is this even a thing?) during the "high phase" just so I can resume working on whatever it is that I am doing at the given moment. This passion for doing what you love regardless of what you are being paid is, among many things, something I highly recommend that you strive for.

"If you are trying to go to the next level, you have to be innovative. Surround yourself with people who are like-minded. I had to build momentum to grow my business fast." Ebony Green, Founder and CEO of CASA Speech and Development Services

The passion for what I do does not mean I don't have a personal life. In fact, being a business owner is what brings me the most flexibility and freedom for a personal life. The flexibility of owning my own business allows me to explore the world ANY TIME I want (Except COVID 2019). I have spent weeks in which I hardly worked; there were weeks I was fed up with my business and needed a break. Traveling is very high on my list of priorities in life; let me be honest, it was a huge reason I chose to work in the public schools when I started my career. Owning a business means I can choose to work in my home office while I raise my children, but the decision was not just based on the children; I am a homebody and an introvert. I have worked from my home or from a "borrowed" home abroad since the start of my business. I can work well in groups as long as I can do so at my own pace as needed.

I can blast Reggaeton music as I work, and I won't be bothering anyone who is coding my next technology or illustrating and designing the next user interface also from the comfort of their homes. I don't have visions of a large castle full of employees, even though that's a very cool idea! That knowledge of what calls my name is what's important to me and what I have already asked you to embrace in previous chapters, and I want you to continue doing it.

I had no idea that running my own business could bring me so much joy because I didn't know this existed. I literally carved this business in the direction that brought me happiness and fulfillment, and in doing that, my business grew under my guidance and was shaped in the exact way I wanted. When I have worked for other people in the past, I was bound by their group culture (in which I may or may not fit in). Think about the mountain of hassle that it takes to change the intake form in a public school district or the many other things you don't feel that you have the freedom to take on in your job because it must pass the eyes and hands of many—although that sometimes is a needed safety buffer. That's why it takes a while for big business to innovate. The bureaucracy would drive me nuts in certain settings.

Starting a business, running it, or taking leadership positions is not for everyone, and that's okay. We all have our gifts. However, I also believe that many of us who were not born into business-owning families can't even fathom the idea that we can go beyond the glass ceiling we just broke by attending college and getting our degree. I'm here to tell you that you can and should experiment with positions and possibilities that you never considered before.

Maybe looking back I can pinpoint many instances in which I was leading. I started a fan club for my favorite music band, became the president of the student council in my college in Brazil, and I was the only one in my class to attend the national speech and language conventions in Brazil as a student; but before starting my business, these were the only leadership roles I actively took. My learning curve was massive, and after twelve years, I am still learning. I am happy that I am learning every day, even when I have moments that I wish I wasn't forced to learn because I ended up having to do someone else's work. That's the downside of being a business owner: you are responsible for everyone's work and everyone's mistakes even when they're not your fault.

I never went to business school, yet here I am, somehow making it. I had to learn about copyright, trademarks, hiring, social media marketing, business tax structures, software development and usability, bookkeeping, and a lot of other things. When you start and manage a small business without an initial injection of funds from investors, which is something I knew I didn't want, you have to wear multiple hats. For many small businesses in niche markets, we will stay small for an indefinite amount of time. In these cases, the owner will have to wear all the hats for as long as the business exists. I still wear multiple hats twelve years into business ownership, and honestly, I love it! Yeah, I may have issues delegating too; but let's keep that between us.

When I started my business, I did the normal things like picking a name, filing with the State of Texas, hiring my first contract developer, and publishing my first apps. Then I started having innovative app ideas one after the other and repeated the process. But you already heard all that. I want to share more details. After all, I am trying to convince you to add to the statistics of female business ownership and innovation in our field and join me.

On any given day, I am managing and chatting with my developers about progress or sharing my brand-new idea for a feature. Then I get on a call with the accounting firm about an issue with the Wisconsin tax office, then I am showing a demo to a school district considering purchasing access for their staff to one of my web platforms, or writing a description about a new app that I am about to release. Every day, I wake up and most of my day is filled with doing things I didn't know I was going to do, and I love this. The readers who use planners would probably lose their minds about the dynamic daily activities of my business life. Don't worry. For many business owners, their daily schedule looks very different from mine; this is what I built and how I operate, and it has worked well for me.

I have many areas in which I still need significant help, even after twelve years in business. I am terrible at marketing and selling what I create. Luckily many of you are awesome at discovering quality products that aren't well marketed, investing in them, or convincing your employer to cover the costs of my products, and that's a big reason why my business flourished and continues to do so. Thank you, resourceful peeps. Our field has built trust in the quality of my apps, and the new products I have created have managed to sell themselves based on that premise. My imperfect recipe is excellence in innovation and product development in a resourceful field.

"Being around people who get things done is inspiring. The year my business started to make some real money, I got a business mentor. Everyone needs a mentor. I actively sought mentorship because I am a small fish in a big pond. I don't have an MBA, and I need guidance from people who know how to get to where I want to go. Being in a group of other women who own businesses was a game changer for me. It made me feel like I had to get to their level." Ebony Green

I am not a salesperson, and businesses need sales in order to grow and prosper. I have yet to achieve the ideal advancements of selling bulk to school districts; which would take my businesses to a new level. So you might think, "Just hire someone, Barbara." Yeah, that's another area of weakness: Hiring. Over time, I have gotten better with my hiring skills by being able to identify quality people more easily in the areas where I have had to do a lot of hiring, such as software engineers and illustrators. Some people may have a talent for it; I have learned this skill through painful hires and fires. However, my attempts at hiring sales representatives have all been a huge and catastrophic failure. That's a current work in progress for me.

Sometimes the power of big businesses has also rained on me in trademark law. I used to have an app called ApraxiaVille. After five years of that app being on the market, I was contacted by the lawyer of a company making a billion dollars a year about my use of the word "ville" and how it infringed on their rights to the name of their Facebook game. Regardless of how much my lawyer and I explained about apraxia of speech and speech therapy, they were irreducible. Ultimately, the cost of lawyers' fees to battle a name with a company that makes billions of dollars was not wise; so I chose to lose all my efforts and costs in marketing for that brand and change the app to Apraxia Farm. While it seems insane that anyone would have the audacity to claim ownership of the word "ville," sometimes it is about making financially wise decisions, and you don't get to fight for what is right or fair. That's a journey I am also still on. However, this experience has taught me that not all fights are worth fighting. Some fights are for someone else to win. All these are experiences I had which completely outside my SLP degree. I am an owner of a technology business with an entirely new set of challenges.

I know that I have made it sound like my life is a wild roller coaster of emotions, learning curves, and curve balls; it truly is. Business ownership is hard. You might be wondering why I am sharing all this bad news and information that is not so flattering about my business practices. Trust me, I debated hitting that delete button many times to delete entire paragraphs of this chapter. However, throughout the book I have shared many vulnerable moments that didn't make others look so good and all the lessons I learned through them. I am also constantly asking you to be vulnerable, and I will have a whole chapter soon about the power of finding your support system completely off of being vulnerable and sharing your struggles. For this reason, I'm willing to be vulnerable too, and I know it will help you. I want you to see that I am comfortable having strengths and weaknesses as I grow my business. When you are intimately involved in the development of sixty apps, all of which focus exclusively on assessing and promoting speech, language, and learning, many of which have been on the top 200 best selling educational apps several times (competing with a staggering number of 500,000+ apps) you develop a sense for what really works and what does not. Nonetheless, I am still looking for support in many places, and this book serves as another platform for my own growth as much as yours. This chapter is merely me practicing what I have been preaching.

This combination of imperfect humanity and imperfect business experiences is how I find myself being my best self. But all of this has led me to another one of my favorite words: Passive Income. Passive income is the reason I have been able to nearly pause all my other activities to dedicate, at times, eight hours a day to writing this book. SLPs around the world are downloading my apps right now. They are signing up for my services, and I am generating income while I am doing something that my heart was called to do. I will receive monthly payments from Apple for the sales of my apps regardless of if I worked today. Of course, this is not a sustainable business practice. I can't not work every day for a year and expect my apps to sell; my business would crumble. In fact, the combination of poorly-developed and cheap apps with neglected app updates is what has led to the downfall and failure of many other speech therapy app developers.

Obviously, not all businesses in our field are passive income businesses. You can start your business by creating physical products that you produce and ship, start your own practice, start your own consulting business, a T-shirt business, a mobile dysphagia assessment business, and many, many others. If, however, you are interested in passive businesses in our field, you could find success in creating your own digital resource for download, a training course in your area of expertise, affiliate marketing, or building and licensing your own software. The most important point is combining things you are good at, things you already know, and gaining awareness of what drives you. The best thing is that you don't have to settle for one; you can have it all. That's what I did, just because I can. You can do it too.

I didn't have much intention of creating a second app when I released the first one. Nonetheless, I have worked on and published over sixty apps on the App Store. I became a paid public speaker on technology and innovation in our field and had the pleasure to travel across the country and internationally. These two accomplishments, in and of themselves, would have been enough to consider myself successful in this field. However, apparently I didn't think that was enough yet. In 2014, five years after I formed Smarty Ears, I formed my second business: Smarty Symbols.

In order to develop apps for Smarty Ears, one of the key components was to either license existing images or create our own. As Smarty Ears grew and the cash flow improved, I progressed from licensing illustrations from random clipart licensing companies to hiring illustrators to create images that would eventually have a specific look and feel that could be connected to my brand. Remember when I shared about my three semesters of photography classes after I finished my master's program? This is where I started using those skills in business. I had enough visual skills and vocabulary to give feedback to the illustrators and designers about the specific aesthetics I was looking to have on my apps.

Around 2011, I started building a library of images that were going to be used in two apps for Augmentative and Assistive Communication (AAC): Expressive and Custom Boards. At that point, I had a need for a symbol library. I had two options; I could license from the existing symbol set creators, which I didn't like for a variety of reasons that I will discuss later on, or I could create my own symbol set library. I hired a team of illustrators, and we got to work. My husband, the English teacher turned Smarty employee, was in charge of creating the word lists and writing the descriptors that the illustrators would follow to create an image that could clearly represent that vocabulary.

The AAC apps were initially released with 500 symbols, and that number grew with each update. Creating my very own symbol set gave me the freedom to also create a variety of language apps using the same images, and it streamlined the development of many other language-based apps. My team was on a roll! As SLPs became familiar with the symbol set within Smarty Ears apps, two other phenomena pushed me to file for Smarty Symbols as new business entity: The growth of SLPs creating their own resources on Teachers Pay Teachers (TPT) and SLPs creating their own speech therapy apps.

They say that rising tides raise all ships. I can confirm that this is true. As SLPs created their resources and were also familiar with the images inside our apps, several of the SLP pioneers on TPT reached out to me, asking for my permission to use my symbols in the creation of their products. The same started happening with other app developer pioneers around 2012 and 2013. In this, I saw an opportunity to build an entire business around licensing my symbols to third parties, and that was the start of Smarty Symbols as a new and separate business entity from Smarty Ears. That's also how people started to call me the Smarty SLP.

Over the years, Smarty Symbols evolved, and the growth speed was much faster than Smarty Ears. After all, at the birth of Smarty Symbols, I'd already had five years of business owning and management experiences. Smarty Symbols was spared a lot of the newbie mistakes I made with Smarty Ears. Today, Smarty Symbols can be found in thousands of downloaded products on TPT by hundreds of SLP entrepreneurs and special education teachers that signed up for commercial licenses with us. Smarty Symbols can also be found in several apps on the App Store and web platforms for education that have partnered with us.

Smarty Symbols grew from a digital library to a powerful web-based platform that is being used by SLPs, SPED professionals, and families to easily create printable visual support materials using our intuitive and modern activity designer. I brought the technology expertise I had with Smarty Ears to build Smarty Symbol's own design builder. A huge win! As businesses, the two Smarties are very different to manage, and as you would expect from someone who thrives with change and variety, I love it. However, one other aspect of Smarty Symbols is a much bigger source of pride for me: Character of Choice.

Smarty Symbols has 30,000 symbols, but what makes it really unique is our Character of Choice. Character of Choice means that we have offered a few character options for the same visual representation when users are creating visual support. More details on that are coming in the **Beyond** section of this book because it speaks to my power to promote change in our field through representation.

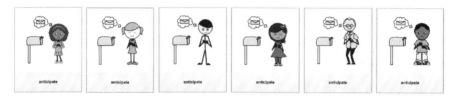

Smarty Symbols - Character of Choice options available

Reflection Question: Can you picture yourself owning a business within our field? What kind of business would you like to own?

Barbara Fernandes

Chapter 18:

From Ideas to Actions and Pivoting

"Opportunities are usually disguised as hard work, so most people don't recognize them." Ann Landers

One of the things that you have heard me say multiple times is to walk through doors when they open, regardless of your fear level. That's what I did again with founding Smarty Symbols. There was an opportunity and a problem, which led to an idea. Opportunities are something that occasionally appear, but often you will have to carve them out. You can't wait for them to be right at your face. Often you have to take action and go find them.

Since I started having booths at the various conventions, I can't tell you how many times I've heard the phrase, "Oh! I had the same idea for an app just like this one." While I do have wonderful innovative ideas, it would be silly of me to think that none of the other 210,000 USA-based speech-language pathologists thought of any of my ideas before. What set me apart was that I didn't stop at the 1% effort (the idea); I put in the other 99% to get the job done. On any given day, you and I have lots of ideas; some great, some not so great. The difference is in what happens after that idea.

In order to scale my business, I could no longer be the only one creating content for all my apps. I started welcoming SLPs who wanted to become app authors by accepting suggestions of apps that they would like to write content for. From that point on, I started to collaborate with other SLPs to create content for the apps I published. I also opened a proposal submission form on my website to give anyone an opportunity to collaborate with me. Our team was flooded with submission ideas. While our team had the capability of tackling several of the submissions, I personally met with many of the authors and gave them instructions on what was needed to go from the idea state to an initial publishing contract with us. 98% of them never got there. As you may know, all Smarty Ears apps are very comprehensive, and in order to achieve that, I required that the authors worked on at least 70% of the content of the app prior to contract signing. If the author had submitted an idea for an app for syntax, for example, I asked them to create target questions and answers on an Excel file. Regardless of the reason, the vast majority of them could not find the time and energy required to create the level of content I required for publishing an app. That's how Smarty Ears stumbled upon a few SLP diamonds who pushed themselves to work on the content of our apps and publish several apps with us: Susan Rosie Simms and Mary Houston, both authors or co-authors of eleven and five Smarty Ears apps respectively. They wrote the content and our team did the technology magic under my supervision.

As you can imagine, if they had not published with us, they would have had even more steps, such as creating a user interface, finding illustrators, hiring voice over actors, and the entire planning and programming process of the apps. That's where I bring out my magic! What I am trying to say is that what separates entrepreneurs isn't necessarily our ability to have ideas but how we go about doing what should come after that idea. Learning to pivot your idea when you see new opportunities or when the business starts to struggle was something I had to learn more recently as well.

As someone who was there from the start, I not only witnessed the explosion of app use in our field, but I believe I was pivotal in that explosion. (I won't be modest here, LOL.) Beyond being the company with the largest and most robust speech therapy app library, I was also training and promoting technology and app use in our field in public speaking engagements and on my blog. I also reviewed apps created by our fellow SLPs.

Unfortunately, as the entire industry became oversaturated with poor quality apps, Smarty Ears also suffered. A failing industry can lead to failure of highly-respected businesses, which is what happened with the SLP app market. The gold rush in 2013 led to an explosion of poorly developed apps. As SLPs started paying for apps that crashed and didn't meet their expectations, SLPs started to become more reluctant in purchasing apps. Many SLP app developers could not financially sustain the constant updates of their apps, which started to crash and malfunction with each new iOS. This environment started to impact my business, and sales started to slow down for us as well. Other factors, such as new devices and trends have also contributed. Today, the market is better and more well-balanced with more quality developers that have remained in business, and my business has since stabilized.

During the shutdown with COVID-19 outbreaks around the world, the demand for my apps saw an increase again. However, this time, clinicians were desperate to learn how to display the screen of the iPad on their computers. Despite GeekSLP's rush to save, the solution was too complex, and there was a desperate need for digital resources that weren't dedicated to Apple devices. SLPs needed a web-based solution. I listened, and that's how I launched my latest Smarty Ears product: **Speech & Language Academy (SLA)**.

Speech and Language Academy is a platform in which SLPs can access all Smarty Ears apps on any device connected to the internet. This subscription-based platform has the potential to become Smarty Ears' most popular product available, and it was born from an existing deficit in the market when it comes to dynamic resources and unexpected global health issues. The quality of telehealth materials available, in my opinion, is to this day subpar in comparison to Smarty Ears' standards. Where there is a need, there is an opportunity. However, it was my ability to react to those needs that led to the creation of my most comprehensive product in our field to date. Speech and Language Academy is also a result of ten years of my contribution to this field through Smarty Ears apps as well as the knowledge acquired from Smarty Symbols in the web-based app development space. Ladies, knowledge is power; remember that! We have to be ready to act when the opportunity appears.

What you don't yet know is that I started developing SLA while I was still in the middle of managing a two-year grant award. Remember that story about the grant that a male colleague didn't believe I could get? Two months after that chat at the TSHA Convention in 2019, a day before I jumped on a plane for a six-week-long trip through Italy and Croatia with my family, I received an email saying that Smarty Ears was awarded a Small Business Innovation Research Award. I remember being so confused, and I almost didn't believe it. My business had its proposal for the development of a new technology for children with either Autism or Hearing Loss funded by the National Institute of Health (NIH) with a grant totaling $225,000 for a period of one year. Based on the written feedback from the reviewers, it was clear that my success with Smarty Ears weighed heavily on their decision. I was the primary investigator (PI) on this award.

"The PI has an extensive track record of bringing communication-related apps to market. Her company is well known in the communication disorders arena." NIH Reviewer #1

"Smarty Ears has a significant track record developing apps for the speech pathology marketplace." NIH Reviewer #2

Never in one million years would I have imagined applying for a research and development grant, much less actually leading a project to be executed at two universities across the country. This was way above my experience level. I literally had no experience managing government funds. I left for my trip ecstatic, knowing that I had a brand-new, exciting project waiting for me to lead when I returned home. Little did I know that the lessons I learned during this award phase would be much more valuable than the award itself.

The project didn't turn out as I would have liked and as I am used to. During the proposal phase, I teamed up with two faculty in the university setting, who introduced me to the SBIR awards. The proposal included a subcontracting award to these universities so that the faculty on the contract, along with paid students, could execute the clinical trial to gather preliminary information about the efficacy of the technology I would create.

The app I created for this project is one of my best works. I am so proud of it! However, I ended up being responsible for activities that were the responsibility and obligation of my research partners. While my primary task was to develop the technology and then hand that technology over for clinical trials, I ended up supervising and training students and doing an incredible number of tasks that not only were not part of my contractual obligations but also way beyond my expertise. Unfortunately, sometimes, even when things are not your fault, you end up having to pick up the slack. As the owner of the business that received the award, making sure the activities got done ethically and responsibly was my responsibility even if it should have been done by someone else on my team. The COVID-19 outbreak didn't make things any easier and prolonged this project for an additional year of commitments. Yeah, business ownership is hard work. I was sitting alone in my office with several iPads on my desk on the evening of December 31st, 2019, testing the accuracy of the audio readings with several decibel readers. All this was way beyond my technical skills, but that's what business owners have to do in order to accomplish goals we set for our businesses. I went beyond my role. I learned. I handled it.

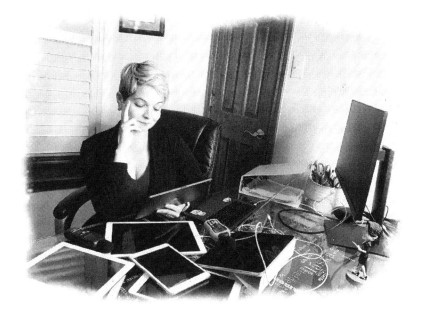

New Year's celebration? This photo was taken at 9 p.m. on December 31, 2019—I was testing an app at my home office desk with seven different iPad models.

Despite experiencing the most frustration of any of the projects I had ever taken on, I learned a lot. I learned because I had genuine connections. There were colleagues in other universities who I could call on, and we spent hours problem-solving the many clinical trial issues I was finding along the way in the process. That's the power of the real connections I asked you to build in this field.

However, here is the best thing that came out of that initial NIH award: while I was developing my technology, the NIH program officer suggested that I apply for another funding called I-Corps. I-Corps awards can be received by NIH awardees in order to learn how to commercialize the technology developed with the original award, as well as test out the market for the new technology; our team received that additional award of $50,000 to participate in I-Corps for six weeks.

During the program, my team of three (me, my husband, and Jackie Bryla) had to interview one hundred stakeholders to learn about their interest level in the technology I had created. We also had weekly classes about bringing a product to market, taught by successful entrepreneurs. Our team was interacting with other participant teams from various health fields. Most of my days were filled with contacting people to interview or interviewing or preparing for the weekly presentations we had to give. Muchacha, this was the most intense program I have worked on; even more than either of my previous educational training programs. However, I felt supported and respected, and the diversity among the participants and instructors created an environment that was productive and collaborative—unlike the environments I experienced in our field. Sis, we can be part of challenging educational experiences and not walk away completely traumatized.

The intensity was not the worst part. After the first week of talking to SLPs, our team came to the conclusion that the stakeholder we had previously identified would likely never buy the technology I had built. When I interviewed parents of autistic children, the feedback was the same. It was not because they didn't find a need for the technology, but because on the list of things that parents and SLPs needed when supporting autistic children, training to listen to speech in background noise was not among the top ten priorities.

I felt defeated. Coming to the realization that the second most incredible piece of technology I had created had no market was difficult. The good news is that as I continued my customer discovery journey, I stumbled upon an entire new segment of the market that I had not considered yet: children with auditory processing disorders (APD). As our team focused our interviews on parents of children with APD, we could see how they understood the need for the technology. The fact that those children rarely receive services in the public schools meant that those parents had been looking for such a product for a long time. It was through this process that I expanded my vocabulary to a word that I had never had to use before: Pivot! Here I was pivoting the technology to match a need in the market. This process taught me a lot about product development and triple checking in with your target audience to refrain from making assumptions about their needs.

I hope all that business info didn't bore you. Here is what I want you to get from that experience: We constantly have to pivot in life. When we don't find use for our skill in one place, we look for a new place. If one group is not interested in what we create, continue to find the group that is. Keep searching, keep adapting, and keep evolving. Often the answer is in our network of people. That's exactly what happened here.

Through this process, I reminded myself about the importance of solving a burning need for whatever solution I was developing. That lesson I learned through my I-Corps experience has already been utilized in major ways at least two times that I can count: creating *Speech & Language Academy* as well as pivoting the use of some of the resources created during the award for some other use in our field.

I had to develop a library of videos of only the face to be utilized in the training sessions for the technology. I hired actors, and for a few days, we recorded them producing a word list that I had put together. The result was a library with thousands of high-quality videos. As this specific technology still required a lot more robust testing for its efficacy, I wanted to make sure that those videos were being properly maximized. Hello, it is COVID-19, and I have a library with thousands of high-quality videos. Let's integrate them into all the articulation and language apps we already have so kids can have models of the whole face—as SLPs have to cover their mouths during therapy. Yeah, brilliant; I know.

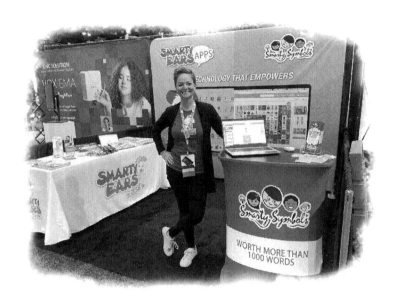

Booth at the 2019 ASHA Convention

I have just spilled a lot of my path in thriving. For me, running my businesses, innovating in this field, and pivoting when my initial plans failed were constant in my life. Despite all the barriers in this field, my background and life experiences continue to bring the best out of me. Resilience, the joy that contributing to this field brings, and my support system have been essential for my success as an SLP business owner, innovator, and leader. Despite the ups and downs of this road and the roadblocks, I know that I have made an impact and left a legacy. I have had the honor of watching SLPs around the world use the products I have invented. I have seen thousands of pictures of my visual support library in classrooms and SLP rooms throughout the USA. This legacy will live beyond my lifetime, and I am so darn proud of it.

I have already done so much, and I am just getting started. Girl, and so are you!

Reflection Question: What aspects of your professional path bring you the most joy?

Chapter 19:

Finding Your People Through Vulnerability

"Vulnerability is the essence of connection and connection is the essence of existence." Leo Christopher

I have already mentioned two of my favorite words: initiative and passive income. Here is another one: vulnerability. I want to tell you how I have grown to find like-minded friends and common ground with colleagues, some of whom became very close friends. It is simply because I have been able to be myself and slowly be more vocal about the struggles of my adventures through life and, in particular, my challenges as a business owner and my experiences as a minority SLP. I have talked about the importance of opening up in many different places in this book, but I find this aspect so important that I wanted to dedicate an entire chapter to it. It is thanks to the fact that my colleagues and friends have made a conscious decision to be openly vulnerable that this book is not just about my journey or my voice. You got to hear their stories of struggle too; and that's why this book became a safe, sacred space not just for me, but for them too.

Part of being vulnerable is having the courage to be who you are without the fear of rejection or prejudice that comes with it, especially when it comes to the parts of you that may be stigmatized by the majority. That's hard. I get it! You don't think I haven't worried about the possible negative repercussions of being so open about so many sensitive subjects in a book, do you? I just opened up a large part of my professional life for you and everyone else to judge. I am scared about the possible email I might get from the people who have a different opinion.

One of the things that my husband has told me that made him fall in love with me is how I have this very lighthearted way of navigating the world. The first time I took him to Brazil, he noticed that my "lightness" was something he saw in many Brazilians he met on the trip. I understood that he was talking about a cultural aspect of my personality that I wasn't necessarily conscious of. If you have been to Brazil, you know exactly what I am talking about. Brazilians are happy, lively, and lighthearted people. We hug and kiss, and we befriend people very easily. Brazilians are extremely informal in their professional life and in college. This will sound crazy to most of you non-Latinx: my whole SLP class in Brazil used to go out dancing or drinking with the faculty of our college as students. Brazilian college students do not call the faculty by their last names either.

As you can imagine, the transition to a more formal academic life was a cultural shock for me. I am a very sensitive, joyful person in my personal life, but for most of my life in the USA, I developed two versions of myself: the professional Barbara who is independent, busy, strong, and fearless, and the other Barbara who is super down-to-earth, informal, lively, sensitive, joyous, adventurous and vulnerable with anyone who wants to hear. That lively Barbara is the Brazilian Barbara. While these two versions have finally merged, it wasn't always like this. Those two versions of me have become one because I have been able to experience the power of my vulnerability and its acceptance from my peers for the other side of Barbara. This personality merge has been a process in the making for a very long time.

At the ASHA Convention in 2017, the day before the convention started, I managed to have some awful blisters on top of my feet. As I explored the shoe section of Target, the only available footwear that I was able to try on without hurting were a pair of white sheep slippers. For the next three days, I walked around the convention center rocking my sheep slippers. I walked as if wearing those slippers had been part of the plan all along. I was comfortable even attending the fancy evening events wearing them. I didn't have an ounce of embarrassment in me. The following year, I bought duck slippers and wore them at my booth. Duck slippers matched my company character much better, after all. This story is a reflection of my entire life: most of the time, bad things happen (blisters), but I "wear" the solution with pride.

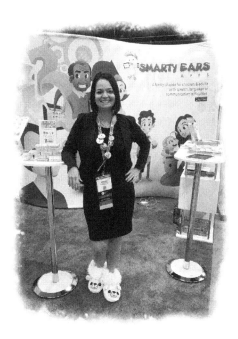

The laid-back, cheerful Barbara that my friends knew at a personal level was showing up professionally. As the owner of my own business, I had the freedom to show up in the world however I pleased. The vulnerability of showing up as myself in a profession that has rejected many parts of me was scary. If my peers rejected me as I was finally brave enough to show up whole, that could have taken a huge toll on my self-esteem. However, as I gave presentations, and felt more comfortable being myself, that joyous side started to appear more frequently as well. SLPs actually really liked that happy, joyful, professional Barbara that starts each presentation session playing fun music. I no longer have to hide that side of me most of the time. The fear of being judged by letting the contributions of my culture shine through my personality has slowly faded.

Vulnerability requires being brave enough to speak up about our professional struggles. These stories of struggle can be about the challenges and fears of entrepreneurship or professional growth or about the experiences that we face as a minority SLP in this field. In this book, I was brave enough to share about both; and in this case, instead of showing people a happy side, I was vulnerable enough to share my struggles. I shared the times I cried, and this made them cry. Finally, they felt seen and understood.

Not all parts of my personality are joyful and upbeat; I have a very sensitive and sentimental side too. The version of Barbara who landed in the USA, beaming with joy and pride, slowly split into two. As my English skills improved, so did my awareness of the more subtle discriminatory behaviors I was experiencing, nearly all in my career. I developed a shield of protection to show up in this new country as the strong one who could keep going and was not going to be taken down by anyone. As I look back at my photographs, I can see and feel the gradual internal change. I trusted no one, and I rarely asked for help because showing that I needed any kind of assistance meant I could not do it on my own. If people were already not believing that I could make it as an SLP, there was no way that I was going to give them a glimpse of my fragilities. I know that I needed that shield, and it was the shield that kept me going strong despite all the feelings and experiences that I have already shared with you. In college, this need to struggle alone may have contributed to the reason nobody was around to help me.

As a business woman, I have often had a poker face that showed things were always great, especially when talking about running my businesses and figuring things out. I have always felt the need to show up strong and confident and hide all the insecurities and worries. I used to go through my experiences quietly. I cried quietly, I failed quietly, and I covered up my mistakes, afraid that they could be perceived as a possible lack of competence. Now look at me, sharing my mistakes and fragilities with more than a handful of people, with literally anyone in the world that wants to know; all they have to do is to get a hold of this book and read. Now I can say I am literally an open book.

"Every time I read my bio or hear it being read out at a conference, I feel a wave of imposter syndrome! A wave of doubt. But why? I earned those credentials! I earned the respect of being an SLP that is sought out to talk and teach about infant feeding. But there is always still a tiny voice within that creates doubt, diminishes what I have worked hard to earn and tells me this isn't real. There is still a tiny voice that says 'don't let your guard down . . . you never know when you'll need plan Z!

Plan Z is what I often say I'm ready for. As an international student, an international worker, and even now as a US citizen, after spending almost twenty-one years living in plan Z, I'm still nervous to let that guard down." Ramya Kumar, Indian American SLP

The tricky question here is: Can we still be perceived as capable professionals when we share our struggles, especially considering that people already see us as the less capable group? Can we still be perceived as professional when we bring our culture into our professional life? I will say, "Heck yes;" but it is tricky. Some of us spent a long time trying to escape the societal stigma that may come with our background or skin color: "too emotional," "too dramatic," "expecting handouts," among others—especially when it comes to cultures that have more public displays of emotions, such as mine. We push through it, building this shield that keeps everyone out. In a field that has the tendency to push us to match the behaviors of the majority, it is easy to associate blending in with the majority or hiding our unique cultural heritage as "being professional." I was not alone either in this conflict:

"It's still difficult, especially as I keep going deeper into the field . . . It's a constant battle of, 'Oh I need to be super serious and always be on top of my game so they know that I am a serious PhD student that should be respected—and as soon as I let loose, they're going to be like, 'Oh, here it goes. A Hispanic girl being silly.' . . . There are times that I feel empowered. That I'm like, 'Yes, I'm Hispanic, I'm from the Bronx, I am spicy, I am loud, I am in your face.' And then there are times that I am just super quiet. 'I just need to listen. The white man is talking or the white lady is talking, and I can't contribute right now because I have nothing to say.'" Michelle Hernandez, Dominican American SLP

"I won't stand up for myself and confront my manager that I deserve to be paid for the extra work I do as a bilingual clinician because I have already been labeled the 'angry Mexican' for standing up for the bilingual families I serve. I don't think I have the courage to show up fully as myself because of this fine line between being assertive or being labeled aggressive." Michelle Posner, Mexican American Bilingual SLP

We want to protect ourselves. The pressure of the stereotypes can make us reserved and quiet. In this process, we become isolated, and being part of a minoritized group is already isolating enough. There comes a time that our protection mechanism no longer serves us, and as humans we want to be able to relate to people. People can't relate to a perfect "professional" version of you. As my professional life evolved, I was able to start healing and merging the two versions of myself into one. I realized that that shield is no longer serving me anymore. That shield was keeping me away from connecting and finding support among my peers.

I want you to start noticing the beauty of the connection that comes with being human and being you while being a professional SLP. This does not happen overnight, but you can start noticing the connections you have made with your close circle of SLPs and how you have built those connections. For me, my most beautiful connections were built because they have known the real me—from the person who saw me cry at the ASHA Convention in 2005 to the person I saw cry at the ASHA Convention 2021, who you will read about soon enough.

My first experience of being conscious about my vulnerable moments was when I wrote my first article about my negative experiences and observations regarding foreign accents in 2010 titled "Nondiscriminatory Standards and Expectations for Speech and Language Pathologists." Since I wrote that article, I have had many articles written about it. I had several students reach out to me asking for advice, and the words I wrote in that article have even been used as an opening statement in a dissertation on the subject. I have connected with several colleagues over the course of a decade because I was willing to start these conversations twelve years ago. Now with this book, I open up about a lot more than that.

Learning to speak up and be vulnerable, when we have been conditioned to shut down, takes time. I spent years learning to suck it up and get it done because I always felt like I had something to prove; and you know how much we feel like we constantly have to prove our worth in this field. However, especially in business, the more I became able to openly share my weak points, my struggles, and self-doubts with other entrepreneurs, the more I could find what I needed: support to continue to grow and to build connections with people who either had similar experiences or knew who I could speak with to get to the next level. For example, I have found creative ways to generate sales for my business from conversations about my poor marketing skills with other entrepreneurs.

Opening up about our vulnerabilities will feel uneasy at first, but it can bring you unexpected rewards, such as developing real, deep connections and healing. I would argue that it is a multi-step process. It is about feeling safe to open up, and that may happen slowly. You can make connections with your colleagues through shared interests or projects, but when it comes to the struggles brought about by our background, that connection can only happen when you have the courage to speak up and be vulnerable. This is because it is only through opening up about our pains and hurt that we are able to connect with others who have or are experiencing similar trauma.

There is so much risk involved in sharing our stories of trauma and pain because we never know if someone will respond negatively or if they will think negatively of us. This is exactly what happened when I opened up for the first time directly to the TCU faculty member that night in the bar about the challenges I faced during my master's program. She rejected my feelings and made me feel as if I had done something wrong by being honest. She validated the idea that honesty in our vulnerability about our experiences is something to be silenced. On the other hand, when I posted a video about that encounter on my social media, the response of support from my peers was overwhelming. In fact, I started receiving messages from my white peers from that graduate program, both apologizing for their inability to be more supportive of me as well as opening up and sharing about their own struggles during the program. It was through their DMs that I learned we had a lot in common despite our differences in background. I admired and respected their courage to reach out to me and be vulnerable as well.

That public display of vulnerability also allowed me to build the connections that inspired me to gather the voices of my minority colleagues who could relate with what I had openly shared and reached out in support through private DMs on Instagram. Through my vulnerability, shortly after an attempt to be silenced, I persisted, and it paid off.

In one of my conversations with PhD student Enjoli Richardson, she affirmed the struggle and reward of choosing to reveal her full self rather than conforming to the expectations and perceptions of those around her.

"I don't have to be led by how others may perceive me. My heart is open because I know that I made the decision for me, and that whatever you're going to receive is fully me and not because I put this on or because I changed my language or I changed my hair . . . I've seen that because I'm stripping away those things that I thought I needed to do, those richer interactions are happening and it is causing other people to feel like we can have a dialogue." Enjoli Richardson

Our vulnerability will eventually shine a bright light on all that we can accomplish despite our trauma, fragilities, and tears. The world hears about our strength to persevere, and we can become a lighthouse for people who find themselves going through the ocean of microaggressions and discrimination and are nearly drowning in sorrow. Eventually, in sharing our stories, we not only find the support we need to keep going; we become the support others need to keep going. The power of that cycle is magical. Sometimes it takes years, but one day, it comes full circle quickly.

The morning of the day that I had the now famous discussion with that faculty member that became the final drop in the bucket pushing me to write this book, something special happened. This experience was the main driving force pushing me to write this book. The experience I am about to tell you about is the magic of generations of women being vulnerable and the cascade effect that it generates. It is almost the end of the book, but here I go with it: Once upon a time at an ASHA Convention exhibit hall . . .

I was at the Smarty Ears booth when I received a text message from Dr. Kia Johnson, one of my closest SLP friends and 2006 MSLP alum, that read:

"I need you to talk to this doctoral student before ASHA ends. I told her to come by your booth."

The text included a photo of a badge with the girl's name. It also read that she was based out of Puerto Rico. A couple hours later, this young girl approached my booth. She was reserved and timidly asked, "Are you Barbara?"

I immediately recognized the name from the photo I had received from Kia, but I didn't have a clue what we needed to discuss. So I asked how she knew Dr. Johnson. Yarimar told me that she was attending one of Kia's presentations, and at the end, Kia asked if anyone wanted to share any comments or experiences as an underrepresented graduate student. Yarimar shared with me that she stood up to thank Dr. Johnson for the encouragement of speaking up and shared with her and the audience that one day, as a fellow clinician, a colleague told her,

"You will never be trusted with your accent as a clinician; be careful."

"Dr. Johnson presented a seminar on strategic mentorship of underrepresented graduate students of color. I was all in tears while expressing this experience to Dr. Johnson and the audience. We had just met. Dr.Johnson replied to me saying that she needed to connect me with 'someone who will help you understand how valuable you are; please go to her now.'" Yarimar Diaz

A few moments later, Yarimar cried in response to me asking about her experiences. At that moment, I recognized that she was the 2005 version of me. Just like me, she was the student who went to talk to the presenter to ask for advice about the turmoil that she was experiencing as a Latina professional with a non-native accent in the United States of America. It was the years of vulnerable accounts about my own experiences that put me in front of that girl who did not yet believe that she could keep going: the girl who was told by her supervisor that her accent was triggering to the families of the children she served. Time froze for me at that moment, and nothing else mattered. We talked, and I shared my journey. I spoke of the gifts I wish she saw in herself. I told her:

"I can see in your eyes that you don't believe me when I tell you how valuable you are as a bilingual clinician. The words used by our colleagues have affected your ability to see your worth. How I wish you could see yourself through my eyes. It will take time because even if part of you believes what I am telling you, you likely don't feel it yet, but please do not give up. I am here for you. Here is my cell phone number."

"I realized at that moment a Hispanic accent does not imply that the person is any less capable. Barbara opened my eyes to understanding that an accent is a gift. She helped me see that a human being like me is smart enough to know two languages and brave enough to do her job in the second. While I couldn't stop crying, I looked at Barbara and expressed to her how out of my comfort zone I feel. I shared about how I have been doing the absolute best to assimilate. At that moment, I was able to see how Barbara could see herself in me. She gave me a hug and support. She provided encouragement and highlighted how much I had already accomplished. My last piece of hope and faith was back. I will never forget November 19th, 2021." Yarimar Diaz

Yarimar's vulnerability connected her with me; her courage to be vulnerable when talking to a stranger she met at an ASHA Convention reverberated and created this domino effect that led to a book. I was only able to be there for Yarimar because when I was in her shoes, another presenter, Vicki Deal-Williams, did the same for me fifteen years ago. In this new cycle, Dr. Kia Johnson and I were the new Vicki Deal-Williams, both shining a light for someone in our field who needed to see her worth. We are four minority women in our field, connected by the power of vulnerability and empowerment. I could only show up for Yarimar because one day someone showed up for me.

Oh, the amazing things that can happen when we speak up. Isn't that such a cliche for us? Let's keep on helping EVERYONE speak up.

Yarimar had no idea how meaningful that moment was for me, and this book is written to tell all the Barbaras and Yarimars of the world:

**Keep going, girl! You can do this, and I am here for you.
Many of us are here cheering you on.**

Chapter 20:

Same but Different

"To Make a Difference, Understand Differences." Syed Sharukh

While writing this book, I learned that even though I could empathize with my colleagues' experiences, I could not help but be alarmed at how much I still had to learn about the different cultures within the culturally and linguistically diverse group. I also learned about the dynamic between some cultures within this group from the other voices in this book. As I heard my peers share their stories, I realized that I was ignorant to some aspects of their journey as individuals of the subgroups that I do not belong to; for example, Asian American. I was also often reminded that we are all unique individuals, regardless of our cultural, ethnic, or racial background. With that, I want to bring awareness to the problem with the big group picture.

It may sound contradictory that I spent most of my book calling for unity among the minority SLPs, but here I am talking about the downside of that unity. However, it is not contradictory at all. The fact that we have been put in this giant melting pot of SLPs can have detrimental effects too, and we need to be aware of it. The diversity within this minority group is too rich for us to not take notice. We would only be reproducing, on a smaller scale, the discriminatory behaviors we feel as minorities ourselves.

We must acknowledge the need to still celebrate the differences among the culturally and linguistically diverse groups and allow the uniqueness of each group to be celebrated. This goes as much for us as we ask of the majority. Accepting the breakdown of minorities in this field might help us understand that there might be groups within that CLD group that are suffering even stronger isolation. I want this awareness to hit you so that you can take actions to reach out and include groups that might struggle to find the power of like-minded colleagues. Take these numbers for example: there are only 0.3% of SLPs who identified as American Indian or Alaska Native; their voices might feel drowned within the larger groups of minorities within the larger non-White. I am asking you to keep this in mind as you go about advocating for the entirety of the non-White group. Groups that make up a larger percentage of the 8.5% need to be attentive to not steal the narrative of the minority groups within the minority group. This could lead to furthering the feeling of isolation for them. We must hold space for our colleagues and become proactive in inviting and welcoming them to have a seat at our table.

Until very recently, I didn't realize that I don't quite fit into any of ASHA's multicultural constituent groups as Brazilians are Latinx but not Hispanics. The group that all the other Latinx SLPs are in is called the Hispanic Caucus. Having a larger Latino Caucus might seem redundant, so in order to include me, they would have to change the Caucus name. Yeah, that's kinda sad and lonely. I have already taken the first step to start a conversation with the Hispanic Caucus to be more inclusive of all countries in Latin America, including countries that do not speak Spanish. But you know what is really cool and very emotional for me? I have always had space held for me among Black SLPs; they embraced me. This feeling of belonging is something I hold as one of the most defining aspects for me as an SLP since the MSLP program in 2006. The space held for me by Black SLPs, and their willingness to include me and make me feel like I belonged in the same places they belonged, was transformative. I have always had space at the table and had my name mentioned in rooms full of opportunities by my Black sisters. I was even invited to give a presentation at their opening session at the NBASLH convention in Washington DC in 2013. They included me. They made me feel a part of, and that's what I ask you to do for someone else within the other less represented groups.

Another side of the same token is that acknowledging the rich differences within the culturally and linguistically diverse group, combined with an awareness of the impact of our culture and our environment on how we see others, means we MUST take active steps in recognizing our own bias toward other minority groups within the 8.5%. We ask that the 91.5% attend the sessions we give at conventions about the bias and challenges of minority students of our own group, but we must be ready to make time to go to the sessions of our colleagues to learn about the bias we might be wrongly holding towards them as well. Are you, as a Black SLP, attending sessions about biases against Asian Americans? Are American-born minorities attending sessions about supporting immigrant SLPs? You have to do what we ask of the 91.5%.

I have become aware that in some cases, I have as much to learn as any of the SLPs who belong in the 91.5% about a subgroup within the culturally and linguistically diverse groups. Thinking that we don't make mistakes and gross assumptions about the experiences of Black, Asian, or Hispanic Americans in this field is detrimental to our ability to support each other and to evolve. Instead, we need to acknowledge that we may also be contributing to perpetuating stigmas about the subgroups within the 8.5% in our profession. I challenge you to ask questions, engage, and be vulnerable about your own lack of knowledge. Stop pretending you know where people are from or assuming that you know about them because you know someone "like them."

> "Achieving cultural competence is a lifelong process that includes self-examination of attitudes originated by what is called implicit biases, your blind spots—a concept associated with unavoidable stereotyping based on preconceived ideas. Understanding the values and needs of others begins with awareness of one's own beliefs and biases. If it's not on the radar . . . then it probably needs to be!
> I keep my hopes of being helpful in the continuing enlightenment and advancement of cultural and linguistic sensitivity in the profession. Diversity opens minds and doors. It makes us smarter!" Maria Claudia Franca, PhD, CCC-SLP, Brazilian American Immigrant

If we want to see change, we must be the change. We can do that by acknowledging that we don't know how others feel and what they are going through. The fact that I am within that 8.5% does not make me entitled to assuming that I understand the struggles of Black or Indigious SLPs in America, for example. I can empathize with a portion of the struggles we share while being cognizant of the fact that I likely have already and will make mistakes and assumptions that will hurt and affect my colleagues. Being a minority doesn't necessarily make you culturally sensitive toward other minority SLPs. Be humble in your acceptance that you might know very little or nothing about some minority groups. Dig deep and ask yourself what assumptions you might have about SLPs of other minority groups.

When people meet me, I know they are curious about where I am from. Some people ask as if they were asking where I bought my jeans. It is a natural question of curiosity; I love it. The same happens when I am speaking Spanish. I love the game I play of having other Spanish speakers try to place where I am from. However, some people, especially since the 2016 election, are too afraid to ask me any questions relating to my background, either for fear of making me uncomfortable or because they are afraid to be perceived as xenophobic. Please go ahead and ask! Be curious; that's how you will learn.

This reminds me of a memorable story I want to share. A few years ago at an ASHA Convention, an Australian SLP colleague joined me and a few friends to go out dancing. She'd flown all the way from Australia to attend the convention in LA. We had no idea where to go, so we asked the taxi driver to take us somewhere fun. He took the four of us to a club in LA, and as we walked in, we stuck out like flamingos among penguins: we were the only non-African Americans in the club. Eventually, we discovered that we had crashed a private party. My Australian friend told me that it had been a dream of hers to be in such a place as she has never had an opportunity to interact with Black people, but it was something she has always wanted to do. African descendants make up only 1% of the population in Australia, and in her geographic region they represent fewer numbers. Her happiness, comfort, and curiosity to learn more about a culture that felt foreign to her was endearing. That's when I realized the privilege I'd had of growing up in Salvador.

I had the honor of attending my friend's Pakistani wedding earlier this year. I was emotional about her cultural traditions during the three nights of wedding ceremonies. I soaked in every second being surrounded by her family and friends. A few of my Latina friends who were also invited didn't attend because they felt uncomfortable wearing traditional Pakistani attire or didn't feel comfortable attending an event that was different from their own cultural norm.

I wish that you and some of my Latinx friends would take a note from my Australian friend's book: break free of your fears. Mingle with people who are different. Feel comfortable wanting to learn more about people who might look, think, pray, or behave differently from you. We should remember that being in the minority SLP group does not give us a blank check of being inclusive and open about other group's cultures. We have to do the work to learn about other groups, accept that we will make mistakes, and go from there.

I will go even a step further; we must also be aware of the diversity within the different minority subgroups. That diversity can be cultural, generational, geographic, or linguistic. Take the Spanish-speaking group, and let me give a perfect example of a real problem with grouping all Hispanics together: assessment items. If you are a bilingual Spanish/English SLP, you know exactly what I am talking about. One of the target items on a famous articulation assessment is "habichuela" (bean). It is difficult to get every child to spontaneously say "habichuela" because in many dialects of Spanish, such as Spanish from Mexico or South America, a different word is used to represent "bean" (frijol). That happens because Hispanics make up a diverse group in and of itself. An Argentinian SLP and a Dominican SLP may have experienced similar discriminatory behaviors for their foreign accent, but each of them has individualities of their culture and dialect that could never be grouped into one larger Hispanic group.

An SLP who immigrated from India as an adult and an SLP who is a second generation Vietnamese American are clumped into the same group of Asian SLPs. Both of them contribute to this group, but I can say that they might have as much to learn about one another as just about anyone else. We must be ready to recognize these differences to avoid making assumptions. This leads me to the following point I want to make: we are all still individuals.

Just as we expect from the 91.5%, we must remember the power of individuality of the people in minority groups as well. It has become common practice for us to use Dr. Stephen Shore's quote, "If you've met one individual with autism, you've met one individual with autism." When we read or even write articles about the whole group, even if we are breaking down the CLD group into subgroups (Asian Americans, Black American, Latinx American, etc), we might end up leading and contributing to stereotypes. As a Brazilian, I have often suffered from the stereotypes of being grouped as part of the larger 6% Hispanic or Latinx slice of pie. In fact, there are a few cultural aspects of being Brazilian that I am ashamed of and have made sure to distance myself from. We are individuals with cultural influences, but our stories are unique.

How delusional would it be for someone to assume that they know you because they have a friend who looks like you or comes from the same geographical region as you? If you met a Black SLP born and raised in Montana, you can't expect that her experiences are the same experiences as a Black SLP born and raised in Washington DC, even though both of them were born in the same country.

Brazil is the fifth largest country in the world, and just like the USA, I came from a country with a large diversity factor. Brazilians born and raised in the northeast, which is the area I am from, have the stereotype of being lazy. There are countless jokes about this floating around the internet. This is also heavily influenced by the implicit bias against the racial makeup of people in that part of the country. When I meet Brazilians who come from states that are considered elitist states, we also battle our very own cultural and even political differences. I am very aware that I can relate better to other Brazilians from the northeast than Brazilians from the south of Brazil. You would do a disservice by grouping people from the same country as one. We are all individuals.

My experiences as a privileged international student coming to the United States with a student visa will be very different from my peer who arrived in the USA as a professional SLP who graduated in Brazil but came to work as an au pair at the home of an affluent family looking for an extra set of hands to care for their children. The fact that both of us are Brazilian accounts for only a portion of who we are and our experiences. We can't expect to be treated as individuals by the 91.5% while at the same time, we, as members of a minority group, aren't willing to allow room for that individuality among people of different groups. Just as you want to be seen for your individuality, be cognizant of everyone's individuality, history, and background.

Finally, in this call for awareness of individuality, I would also like to ask that you acknowledge that the 91.5% isn't a homogenous group either. We must respect the diversity that comes from that group in all the same aspects: their history, their background, their environment, and their willingness or lack thereof to learn and do better. We can't expect them to do better when we aren't willing to teach, answer questions, or speak up. Once we do speak up and share, then they can decide, as individuals, if they will null our voices or move into a state of awareness. It is their individual choice, just as we can choose to see them as an individual. They will be asking questions, and we should be able to make our own decisions on how we want to go about sharing our stories.

Reflection Question: What is something you wish people better understood about how your culture differs from the larger minority group that you belong to?

Barbara Fernandes

Chapter 21:

Different but the Same

"One of the greatest regrets in life is being what others would want you to be, rather than being yourself." Shannon L. Alder

This is a chapter about unity. We can't thrive without it. We can't thrive without the awareness of the likeness of our stories or the awareness of behaviors of exclusion from within. We need to acknowledge that our minority SLP colleagues are worthy of their own opinions, behaviors, and choices even when they are different from our own. Differences of opinions and choices in our field shouldn't create separate groups. We have a lot of work to do both on ourselves and as a group in order to move the needle of injustice in the right direction. This is the chapter where I ask you to give grace and belonging to your minoritized colleagues who may not be like you, agree with you, or act like you. That's not an exercise I did until recently in many aspects of my life on earth. As we blame, shame, and oppress from within, we shift the focus from what matters the most.

When I think of controversial topics and about having controversial conversations, I love thinking about achieving common ground as a starting point; we have common ground with women who do not belong in the minority group when it comes to the disproportionate number of men in leadership roles in our field. You have seen through a few of the stories I have shared in previous chapters that while the minoritized group is diverse and even though we are all unique individuals, our stories share a lot of similarities. When I decided to write this book, I asked my colleagues to either write and send me their stories or to schedule a Zoom call with me. The Zoom call slots were sometimes booked for fifteen to thirty minute durations; however every single one of them lasted *at least* one hour. That means we spoke for at least double the amount of time we thought we would. At some point, I was aware of that gap in duration and adjusted my calendar accordingly. As I listened to their stories, we kept discovering topics and areas that we had in common, so the conversations were prolonged each time. We cried in nearly every single virtual meeting. I had so much in common with every single one of the contributors of this book that I felt them. During those calls, I experienced a range of emotions: not only anger, frustration, and surprise, but also pride and connection. That's empathy.

I spoke with Black SLPs born in the USA, immigrant SLPs, second generation Hispanic SLPs, Asian American SLPs, single mother SLPs, business owners, students, and so many other SLPs. While we all have unique experiences, I could feel every single one of their words as if they were coming out of my own mouth. As a group, we had our own colleagues attempt to crush our dreams and self-esteem. We went into depressive states, we felt oppressed, and we let the words of the majority and their microaggressions consume our souls. In a way, most of us are still learning to navigate this field. I know for sure, now reaching the closing chapters of this book, that I have had enough of this bullshit, and I know that I am not alone. From the SLP who grew up in the Bronx to the Brazilian immigrant, unity is the only way. You have witnessed the power of the numbers that the 91.5% have in getting awards and advancing white men into positions of prestige, and I want you to round up and support your sisters, girls, amigas, and muchachas in any place they are. I want you mentioning their names in moments of glory. Save their seats next to yours.

Regardless of how unique we are, the vast majority of the voices that contributed to this book still share similar heartbreaking stories navigating this field, and that is something we need to be paying attention to. I want to share a few more of my observations as I spent hours either reading through the submissions of stories I received for this book or listening to the stories of our colleagues through our virtual meetings.

At the start of each chat, I would tell them to share anything they wanted regarding the subject of my book. As I listened to a highly summarized version of their journey, or a highlight of a phase of their lives, I had to control myself every time I heard stories that related to mine. Something I learned from my own therapist was to let people get things off of their chest and not interrupt them. So, I listened and kept notes about every time our hearts connected through similar soul-crushing experiences and tried to bring them up when I could feel that each one of them got to a point in which they felt done. Hearing someone share an experience that so closely resembles mine and not shouting #meTOO, girl, was one of the hardest things I did in this process. I realized that I was not listening with my ears; I was listening with my heart.

All the voices you heard through this book shared grit and resilience, which I believe is transformational in many ways and has the power to shape us into better versions of ourselves. There was so much overlap in the stories I heard that at times I found myself screaming silently, "Girl, I KNOW!" as I let them share.

"I wear the bilingual badge buddy at work. I went through a verbal test and qualified to be a Hindi interpreter. The company did not have a test for the other Indian language I speak, though. The number of times I get asked to interpret in Spanish is crazy, and I always have to say, 'There are many other languages in the world that you can be bilingual in.' It has definitely irked me, but I think that defense mechanism made me brush it off like Teflon here too." Ramya Kumar

As an SLP whose first language is Portuguese but who had to learn Spanish in order to have my language skills count as a "bilingual SLP," I can absolutely scream here too, "I know, girl, I know!"

Another one of the recurrent themes was the doubt in our capacity to thrive and the constant doubt in our professional judgment.

"There was silence and quick acceptance when I expressed my desire to discontinue my PhD program." Phuong Lien Palafox, MS, CCC-SLP, Vietnamese Chinese

"'No, Michelle, you don't really know what you are talking about. Let's hear what John Doe has to say,' said my evaluator coordinator when I tried to explain a procedure about bilingual assessments to him. I was there for ten years. I knew what I was doing, but he preferred to hear from someone who had been there for only one year who was white and male." Michelle Posner, Latina SLP

These spaces, faces, and voices make us feel inappropriate, incapable, and isolated. We hear messages that perpetuate a lack of belonging everywhere. Unfortunately, these messages are also coming from minoritized SLPs themselves. Many of our minority colleagues are afraid and discouraged enough. We need to take a closer look at how we might be adding to their feelings of unworthiness, inappropriateness, or inadequacy ourselves. We can't expect our clients to keep improving and keep pushing mastery of hard skills if we keep shaming them for not trying hard enough. I know you don't do that with them. Let's stop doing this to ourselves. Being accepted for who we are is the basis of belonging. That's what we want for everyone. Let's start acting accordingly.

I love social media. It has allowed me to thrive and have a voice. It is a place where many of us have been able to start experimenting with speaking up. As we gather the courage to speak up, we must also have the awareness to be accountable for how the words we use make others feel; especially how we make our own girlfriends, who already struggle so much with injustice and isolation feel. As I navigated some social media accounts of minority SLPs tackling similar subjects, a few comments and post descriptions caught my eye and consumed me for several days. Many posts and comments come across as if we were in an Olympic game to see who qualified as a "minority." The separation I felt reading comments toward other minority SLPs as not worthy of belonging to the group was saddening. Their profile photo, their background, their workplace, and even previous job titles were all used to determine their worthiness to be in the "minoritized" group as if one person's pain was less real than the other. While I agree that there is a privilege that comes with "looking or acting" less minoritized, excluding people from a seat at our table is inflicting the same pain you felt from the 91.5% on others. As I tried to understand, these posts or comments were often directed toward people who were struggling with oppression too. These posts were insinuating that an oppressed SLP who has achieved so much in the field could not possibly relate—or worse, be trusted. This created a separation that we can't afford. The verbiage is being used in the SLP social media sphere to push down people for not being Latina enough, Black enough, Asian enough, or for not having a stigmatized enough accent or a challenging enough background. My heart ached for those women, and I would like this group to be a group of acceptance and tolerance, not of division.

A group of speakers with a foreign accent perceived as "strong" claiming that the group of speakers with an accent perceived as "not strong" is facing a lot less discrimination and their experience can't be valid is, in my opinion, a waste of our own energy to promote change. The nuances of discrimination are complex and often determined by the perception of each person making the racist or xenophobic remark. Racism and discrimination happen in a context. A person with a barely distinguishable foreign accent in our field might experience one hundred times more discrimination than someone with a strong influence of their native language in English in a field such as engineering. The context of the oppressor impacts people differently. The same goes for work environment, area of focus, or the person's geographical location. It may even have no relationship to what the accent even sounds like. This is not a competition for validity. Our focus needs to be on our shared experiences against those minoritizing ALL of us. Nobody should hold qualifying checklists to belong in our team.

We cannot make changes by pushing our own people down just so we can feel empowered. We are barking up the wrong tree when we start accusing other minorities of being less deserving of the "minoritized" status. We need each other! Unity, ladies! If you have been made to feel less worthy by your minority colleagues, I am sorry you were made to feel inferior from within. You belong here!

Acceptance and tolerance have also been lacking among us when the topic of race and ethnicity have been brought up in SLP social media spaces. Unity does not mean getting people to think and act like you. We have been demanding diversity of thought from the 91.5%, but somehow, some have expected that a diverse group think in unison. There appears to be a huge divide between minority SLPs who have been involved in one or more of the multicultural activities promoted by their state associations or ASHA and the ones who feel abandoned, unheard, and neglected by the association. There are minoritized women who do not feel they can talk among themselves, engage in a discussion, and listen to the other person's side without fear of being an "ASHA suck up" or "ASHA hater." Both sides feel targeted. Both sides want progress, but both are unable to listen to and communicate with each other. I have personally heard and read comments such as "the token Black SLP who does anything a white person at ASHA tells them to." It made me sick to my stomach as I watched some of my fellow minority SLPs and close friends being accused of not thinking or acting for themselves. Enough! We can't thrive without tolerance, support, and grace for our own fellow minority SLPS.

Minority SLPs are being judged even for staying silent. I have myself remained silent in some online discussions because I felt like I could not disagree or bring up points to consider. I have stayed silent if I didn't feel I had enough information to formulate an opinion. I have stayed silent if I had too much happening in the many other areas of my life. I have stayed silent if I just didn't have the energy to make a post or a comment. Enough judgment already! In one of my moments of silence, an SLP colleague from the 91.5% felt that it was appropriate to question my silence directly in a private message on Instagram. She had no idea what I had been doing or how I had been working behind the scenes, but even if I just wanted to take a chill pill, I should have been able to do so without feeling judged or pressured to do anything. Yeah, a woman belonging to the majority will judge a woman belonging to the minority on how/if/when she shows up for others in the minority group. I don't want to have that same type of judgment from you, though. Now, it would be extremely hypocritical of me if I expected a voice from everyone, yet I chose to remain silent myself. That's a whole other story. But as I said before, for various reasons, let's stop throwing the baby out with the bathwater. If people have been supportive for twenty-nine days of the month but stayed silent one day, why focus on that one day!? Enough already! Let's trust that each of us can be responsible for our own decisions and actions.

We've created our very own suppressive culture among minority SLPs, and that's alarming. Some of us already have fears of speaking up about our own experiences; we don't need to suppress differences of expression when discussing our own issues.

I am watching division among minority SLPs unfold in front of my eyes, all because we either failed to gather more information, listen to different arguments, or accept and respect different opinions. Differences of opinions do not make us less capable of empathy and connection. Enough with that already!

Online is not the only place where I have witnessed or experienced firsthand the impact of this lack of unity. Throughout this book, I have been writing rave reviews about how my Black SLP colleagues embraced me and made me finally have a place to belong. As that was happening, I was experiencing a reversal situation at my workplace at the public school in the Dallas Metroplex. Given the demographics of the area, most of the staff were Latinx professionals who did not make the only Black SLP feel welcomed. They did not give her a place to belong. I didn't do enough to bring them together. As the "traveling SLP" who was often in a different building each day, I heard most of these accounts secondhand long after. I often found myself in the middle of their many conflicts on what felt like a clear clash of cultures, with the Latinx staff being emboldened by their numbers, ready to blame her at every turn. That tension was so full of biases, and I, as an uneducated empath at the time, didn't have the tools or knowledge to intervene; but I felt the impact of the crossfire of emotions. As I look back at that exclusion, I might have been too young and unprepared to have intervened. However, I wish that despite being young, someone had already brought up these topics for me to think about and feel prepared and ready to bring them together. I failed my Black coworker. I wish they could have found a sense of togetherness in 2008. We are on the same team, ladies. I reconnected with her in 2018, and I was able to support her the way I know best: giving business mentorship and promoting her business. This is a story for yet another call for unity. While I was unprepared in 2009, you are not anymore.

No level of professional success will be enough for you to not feel the hurt of being left behind. I have even recently felt the impact of this lack of unity. A minority colleague, with whom I worked on a project, wrote an article to talk about a new technology she contributed towards. She failed to mention that the idea for that technology was mine. She failed to mention that I, alone, created the entire content for the app. She failed to mention that I was the leader of the project with my team at Smarty Ears. In fact, my name was not mentioned at all in the article. She would not have been doing me any favors; she would have simply been telling the truth. I felt left behind as she chose to only acknowledge our white collaborator, whose contribution was, at best, minimal. I can't say that her choice of whom to acknowledge wasn't an indication of who she perceived as holding more decision-making power. Unfortunately for all involved, she was wrong. I still hurt too. Regardless of how high we climb, we still need each other. We, aware of the barrier we face, should always remember to keep a seat at the table for each other.

I know that we may argue innocence for being pushed to follow the masses. We are often fighting to survive in this field and it may lead to picking up a flag to wave that we might not have picked up if we had just known a bit more-if we had taken a few more moments to gather our thoughts and information or make inferences and reach conclusions or just to take a breather. It is also possible to say that we have become prone to be hyper-critical as a "woke" society. It almost feels as if it is our job to complain, accuse, and be cynical to make us look or feel empowered. I say this fully aware that this entire book was my own attempt at being "woke." I have thrown several of these cynical concepts at you with thousands of words previously. I am aware of it. This process is necessary for progress. However, it does not need to be done without attention and care for the same behaviors we wish weren't upon us every step of the way in this field. Let's break the cycle.

We are all in this together.

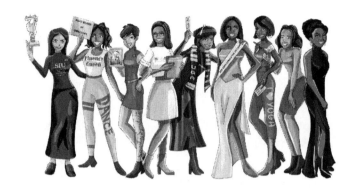

Part Three: **Beyond**

Chapter 22:

Representation that Inspires

"It can be difficult to speak truth to power. Circumstances, however, have made doing so increasingly necessary."
Aberjhani, *Splendid Literarium: A Treasury of Stories, Aphorisms, Poems, and Essays*

Given all that I shared previously, it seems that the next logical step in this book would be to answer the question: How do we make things better for everyone? How do we make sure that if our daughters decide to follow our footsteps and become SLPs, the barriers they face will not be as tall as ours? How do we make sure that future generations of SLPs don't feel so alone? As somebody who has avoided confrontation, and still does, ruffling some feathers is never my intent. However, I found myself unintentionally doing just that at the 2021 ASHA Convention. Writing a book to tell my stories was not my first instinct, but here I am. My first instinct is doing things in the way that fits my personality. While writing a book was not part of it, doing it in twenty-eight days is.

This book was not written to enlighten whatever portion of the 91.5% needs to do better; I will leave that book for you to write. This book was written for you: the minority SLP. That means I will be sharing some thoughts on how you can take the driver's seat to promote the changes we so desperately need in this field. One of the things we desperately need to give others is hope.

Minority SLPs are walking billboards of inspiration and hope in and of itself. I know that nobody walks around with the goal to inspire others. It is a consequence of living a life that speaks to your truth. My niece, Larissa Fernandes, who lives in Brazil, was inspired to become an SLP. I didn't become an SLP to inspire her. It happens naturally. Just earlier this year, she received her diploma and became an SLP and Audiologist in Brazil. Inspiring her was not intentional. She just saw that I was living the life of my dreams in such a rewarding field. You are inspiring people every day, and you might not even know it yet.

Don't get me wrong. I am grateful that I have friends and colleagues taking on the journey to speak up, demand change, be the change, and get involved in professional organizations. They are not just talking the talk, they are walking the walk with actions, time, and energy to promote progress in this field. I hope they know that they are inspiring others but not only by their actions—they inspire just by being there. They inspire others by being the first ones and by appearing on fancy photos on websites. I see them making up 30% of ASHA's 2021 board members. Their black or brown faces, their unique facial features, their culturally-influenced personality, and their poise and grace inspire more of us to aim for that space. I hear them speaking at opening sessions, closing parties, and the many fancy ASHA events. I applaud them, and I get emotional seeing them go places because I know everyone else sees it too. There is so much value in inspiring others just by living your amazing SLP life in your skin with your own traits. As clinicians, we can inspire the children we serve, their families, or our own colleagues simply because we exist. It is through inspiration that we can become the catalyst for change. You are someone people are looking up to.

Inspiring minority kids to become a new generation of future SLPs is worthy enough. As you sit in your chair, bean bag, or on the floor supporting their learning and growth, they look up to you. At that moment, you can become the catalyst for more diverse children to earn their CCC-SLP one day. Some of you may be too young; some of you might have already experienced this. At times, that inspiration starts even earlier, with the parents of the children we serve as clinicians.

The first time I experienced the emotions of the power of representation was during my transition between my full-time job at the public schools and my full-time role with Smarty Ears. I worked two days a week as a home health evaluator for bilingual (Spanish/English) children. During one of my home visits, the mother was ecstatic to see me come in. She shared that she was apprehensive about the evaluation due to the fact that she communicates better in Spanish. However, she never expected an SLP who spoke Spanish.

After I finished the evaluation, the mother of the child demonstrated a particular interest in how I had that job. She seemed surprised and at the same time proud of me. We had just met, yet she saw her own child's opportunities through me. She said, "I am so happy to see you today. You weren't even born here, but you went to college, and you are now a **_therapist_**!?" Here, she emphasized the word "therapist" in such a way that she made me feel as if I had just achieved the highest office in the land. She continued, "If you did it, I know my child can get there too!" I remember that day as if it was yesterday; I had goosebumps.

As I walked out of that home to write my report, I felt incredible! I connected with that mother, and I almost walked her through the application process for college in the USA for her three-year-old child. As a recent immigrant, she didn't know anyone in her circle who spoke Spanish and had a professional degree. She was afraid that by speaking Spanish to her child, she would hinder her child's ability to learn English and eventually go to college, to which I replied, "Mom, listen. I am getting paid more **_because_** I speak English and Spanish. Keep speaking Spanish to your child. That's your gift to her."

Pang Tao Moua, PhD candidate, shared about the importance of representation in making therapy an option for everyone. Relatability and understanding of their culture was something extremely important for Pang's family.

> "My grandfather had a stroke and was struggling with aphasia. It was really hard for our family to combine our Shaman beliefs with western medicine, and it was hard to find someone, like a minority SLP, to understand where we are coming from to convince my grandfather to receive therapy or to convince my family to pursue rehabilitation. When I saw that gap in our field, that's when I decided that I wanted

to pursue speech and so hopefully other minority families don't go without receiving therapy because they can't find a therapist that they can relate to." Pang Tao Moua

At times, our professional connection to families is one of linguistic and cultural representation, making parents feel seen and understood. In fact, Pang has already been able to provide the exact feeling she was looking for during her own experience in one of her externships:

"When I was working on my internship at an acute care hospital, I was assigned a Samoan patient. I am not Samoan, but for her and her family to see me as another person of color, it was a magical experience for them. I could see it in their eyes! They felt that I could understand them because I look like them. It is almost as if my background helps them relate and feel understood. There was an underlying cultural connection even though I don't know much about the Samoan culture; I could feel their happiness when they saw me. They kept saying, 'She gets us!'"

This connection can be even deeper when there is both a background and linguistic connection, as Phương brilliantly shared with me:

"She held my hand with such strength under the table as the teacher spoke during the IEP meeting. I felt our first meeting just minutes prior, albeit brief, held such power and comfort. Her eyes shone when I walked into the room. 'Cảm ơn, cô Phương. Thank you, Ms. Phuong,' she repeated every few sentences. I was the first Vietnamese educator she had met during the years her fourth-grade son attended school. With her first glance, words and tears poured from her. We had a mutual narrative, and it buoyed her understanding of complicated processes within the schools. More importantly, I gave her permission to resume the lovely tones of her native Vietnamese with her child—something she was (erroneously) directed to discontinue when he was three years old so 'he wouldn't be confused.' I honor the power of all languages of influence. I am thriving." Phương Liên Palafox, Vietnamese Chinese Bilingual SLP

The next layer of the inspiration of representation is the one that had the most impact for me: being an example to younger minority SLPs. Guiding them, becoming a mentor, or simply walking your nice self through the convention center during any given conference and making your presence be seen by everyone.

My work style and entrepreneurial spirit has never been compatible with participating in the formal mentorship program at ASHA. However, for years, I have been a type of word-of-mouth promoter of ASHA's MSLP program. I have done that at my booth or as I walked through the exhibit hall and met other minority SLP students. I can't count the number of times that I have told students:

"Open the notes on your phone, write this name, 'Minority Student Leadership Program,' and look it up tonight. Put on your calendar the due date to apply. Trust me on this!"

I know that I have done this at least two dozen times since 2006. In fact, this year, I was at a night event at ASHA when someone approached me and said, "You are the Smarty apps lady, right? I met you the year you were wearing slippers, and you told me to apply for the MSLP program. Can we take a photo?"

My contributions are not through the traditional route, but it is my style. You just have to find yours too. My colleagues who are always volunteering at the national or state level associations have tried to convince me to do it their way. It has not worked thus far. It does not matter if you become directly involved at NSSLHA, ASHA, NBASLH, or one of the caucuses or if you simply go around the exhibit hall telling strangers to not give up and keep going. Sis, do you! Just like Phương Liên Palafox does:

> "As I sat down to write this piece at 9 p.m., my phone rang. When she calls, I always try to prioritize her, a Vietnamese-American speech-language pathology graduate student. I remember not seeing anyone who looked like me when I navigated a system that my family had no understanding of. I remember the loneliness. So, I pick up. She shared

her ache. She shared her family's sacrifice to pay for her education. She shared her doubt. There's so much doubt. I quit my doctoral program, and no one told me that I was needed in the program. Not a single person was in my corner to say, 'I know. I KNOW you can do this, and you are so NEEDED in our space.' I speak honestly to her. 'How I wish you could see the version of you that I see and feel.' I tell her that we need her gifts and her stories. We hang up, and I feel hope for our future because of her. *I provide the empowerment and support that I wish I had. I am thriving."*

Phương's recount of the support she gave this graduate student nearly mirrors the support I gave to the PhD student who came by my booth at ASHA just a month ago. We are able to hold space for these young women because we finally found our worth, and we can see the value they will bring into the field with an impact that only we can give.

My Brazilian SLP niece and I are very close. As much as I would like to have her in the US, I am not fully convinced that I want her to have her soul crushed by pursuing a master's degree here. Unfortunately for her, it still takes a lot more than dedication for an immigrant to earn a CSD degree in this country. Thankfully, this is not everyone's experience. Have hope, please. Through this process, I learned that a few of us had incredible experiences heavily influenced by the power of representation.

"In 2001, I was an SLP faculty with a master's degree in Brazil and received a small scholarship to visit a few universities in the United States. In this process, an opportunity appeared for me to become a teaching-assistant while I pursued a PhD followed by another master's program at the University of Southern Illinois in order to receive my certificate of clinical competence (CCC). My experience was extremely rich, and today I am still at the same university where everything started, now as an SLP faculty member. The University mission for promoting diversity and supporting international students was pivotal. You can find foreigners and minorities everywhere you go on campus in positions of leadership, including the chancellor and the provost of the university. I have always felt welcomed and supported as a multicultural SLP because my experiences were empowering, and I was surrounded by diversity." Maria Claudia Franca, PhD, CCC-SLP, Brazilian American SLP

Dr. Franca's account of feeling empowered and safe as an immigrant in her university environment validates the importance of representation in positions of leadership. She shared with me that several university colleagues have been able to experiment with international collaboration with other Brazilian universities through her initiatives; many faculty have even visited Brazil to collaborate abroad. Dr. Franca is planning on taking her first group of students to Brazil this coming summer to broaden their education in international issues within our field.

Maria Claudia and I met at the MSLP program in 2006. We have remained close friends and colleagues for the last fifteen years. Through her presence, Maria Claudia is serving as a beacon for other SLP immigrants, but she is going above and beyond by promoting change through awareness to hundreds of students who have gotten to learn from her over the years. Maria Claudia amplified her reach, visibility, and impact by becoming the president elect of the Illinois Speech and Hearing Association (ISHA). Go girl!

Maria Claudia's representation in this profession as an immigrant with a non-native accent as the president of ISHA matters; but she is going beyond representation. She is taking an active role in leadership in this field, and as a result of that, we will all rise with her. Don't get me wrong, representation does matter a lot. I just spent two pages in this book telling you the power of representation and how much we inspire just by doing us. It is not cliche. I am living proof of it. Your representation as a minority SLP is valuable in and of itself. You are walking proof that your accent, your skin tone, your hair, and your background did not hold you back. Yeah, most of us had to climb taller mountains, but we did it anyway. May you one day experience what I have been blessed to experience in hearing that you have inspired people just by the simple fact that you exist.

The third layer of the power of representation is the one that shows the people who don't believe people like us are actually capable of or should be doing things like what I am doing. The faculty who said that my accent was a communication disorder, the one who told Pelesia Fields that she was not cut out for this field, the SLP who didn't think I stood a chance at winning an NIH award, or the the many other naysayers can now open their iPads and download one of my sixty apps, see my symbol set used by their students, or buy this book to read about all that I have actually achieved. Yeah, all of that has a nice, sweet taste of victory. I wonder if they will think twice before doubting the capacity of the next Latinx student who applies to their program. Honestly, I am not fully convinced of it. Nonetheless, let me be clear: you do not have to be a role model for them either. Be you. Do you. All else falls into place.

With all that said, I used to think that just being a good role model of a minority speech-language pathologist was enough for me—but what does being a role model even mean, anyway? Aside from being awesome at being ourselves and inspiring other minority SLPs to reach for the stars, what does it mean in everyday examples? Does it mean going to college, getting good grades, completing your work, being compliant and ethical, attending ASHA Conventions, doing more than your fair share of work quietly, giving a fake diplomatic answer about your journey, silently listening to sexist or ignorant comments? Maybe it means acting and behaving in a way that tones down who you are so you can fit in? I don't think so . . . which is why I say again: Be you. Do you.

I used to believe that when my colleagues saw me thrive and achieve, or when I became a walking example of what people like me can do, their perception of people who are like me would have the trickle-down benefit. Unfortunately, that is not enough. I had risen to a position high enough to be able to show a white, male SLP that regardless of his perceptions about immigrants, people with accents, or minorities, I was his boss—I was hiring him, and I was assigning him tasks. But I am still a woman with what he called a "not so bad" accent. Based on what I have shared in this book, my achievements were not enough for me to have respect that day, and they weren't enough for my minority SLP sisters. I needed to do more than be a walking, living, and breathing example. I was inspiring others, but I needed to promote real change.

Reflection Question: Do you also feel a need to do more than inspire?

Chapter 23:

Promoting Change

"No voice is too soft when that voice speaks for others.**"**
Janna Cachola

In a field where minorities are underrepresented, the logical next step might seem to be to attract more minorities to this field. ASHA has made significant attempts to recruit minorities in the last few years. However, I would argue that we need to focus on the retention and graduation rates of minorities first. Focus on promoting a work environment that is safe for minorities. Bridge the communication and information gap between the majority and the minoritized so that everyone knows what is appropriate in a peer level situation.

Why recruit us if we will be pushed to drop out of school or to abandon the field? Not to mention how undergraduate CSD programs are leaving many of us behind with only a bachelor's degree and student loans, rejected from master's programs. The ones who survive end up traumatized. The goal has to go beyond inspiring young men and women to apply for the programs. Before our field can recruit more students, we must first acknowledge the desperate need for our field to support the ones already here.

When we are faced with reminders of our own pain, we want to take an active role in bringing about this change. That's exactly what happened to me. I wanted to give hope to SLPs on the verge of giving up. When I think of all I heard and read through the voices in this book, it felt pretty obvious to me that things must change, not only in our education path, but also in our workplace. Microaggression, bias, isolation, xenophobia, racism, and sexism can be found everywhere; these are not exclusive behaviors of our profession. As much as we have seen a huge push for cultural sensitivity and compassion within our field toward our clients, minority SLP students and professionals still don't have the same peer-focused training. We don't have a structured safety net in CSD programs. A profession that, by its nature, should be more accepting of diversity among its students and professionals still has far to go in this aspect.

I am not talking about the diversity acceptance rate or diversity hire. I am referring to real support that understands and values students and professionals who can provide a unique point of view as we drive this field forward. With an understanding of this value, institutions will create an environment of acceptance—an environment in which we can thrive and be ourselves.

I am not the most qualified person to discuss execution plans for academia changes. However, I am great at having unique ideas; I am an innovator, remember? I am sure that among the folks reading this book, a few of you will say, "I know how we can go about putting this idea into action," and you will do it. We all have different personalities, which will lead to different paths of action. There are many changes, though, that do not require any specific or elaborate master plan. They require a shift in attitude.

Connect with your minority peer or colleague. If you are fortunate enough to have another minority student in your program, go ahead and engage! Share your struggles. Be willing to be vulnerable. You may not be ready to be vocal yet to a faculty member or your boss, but open up to your peers, exchange struggles, and support each other. There is power in sharing and connecting. It gives both of you a sense that you are not alone. You don't have to become best friends; after all, we are all unique individuals, and there is a lot more to us than our background. If you are a student at a larger university with students of different levels or different years in the program, extend your reach to those who are earlier in the process. I remember feeling so out of place that the idea of participating in the National Student Speech Language Hearing Association (NSSLHA) chapter along with my white peers felt so foreign. I believe I never quite even understood what it was until I became a professional.

Obviously, given the percentage of minorities entering this field, most of us will still be in classes with a majority white student body. That has not been the biggest issue. Non-Hispanic white people are still 61% of the US population, according to the 2013–2017 American Community Survey (USCB, 2018). That's okay. We are looking for acceptance and support so that despite being the minority number, we will no longer be minoritized. Could I have found a support system if I had opened up more? I don't know. Here is what I do know: through this process, a few of my peers from college reached out to me. Some related to my experience in a different way, and one wrote, "Wishing I could have supported you better." I understand that many of them couldn't possibly have known what I was going through because we never became close enough for me to open up. As young women in our early twenties, which is the age most of us go through CSD programs, many of us still had limited life experiences. Some of my classmates were meeting a foreigner for the first time in their lives. They never mistreated me, but today I wish they knew more about me. I wish I had opened up more. But as we scream to be seen, sometimes we are already drowning and it is too late for positive interactions and support—which is why I want to brainstorm proactive solutions. I want you to be brave. I want you to open up. Give others a chance to support you.

I keep brainstorming how to solve this lack of support problem. Not everyone has an amazing professor who will take us to another country through a study abroad program or help us be more sensitive toward cultural differences. In fact, when universities do these study abroad programs, often only the bilingual students take part in them anyway. We can draw from solutions that have worked. As an international student, both at Temple and at TCU, we are supported by an international office. There is an orientation that discusses American culture, myths and truths, and expected behavior for interactions with professors, among other things. What if we turned the tables? Wouldn't it be great if we could create a similar cultural sensitivity training for all CSD students as part of their orientation at the start of the program? What if the dominant group learned how to support the minority students?

At some point in my life, I decided that I was going to adopt children from the foster care system. In order to obtain a license to adopt, the adoptive parent must complete a series of trainings on trauma and the adopted child. In Texas, parents must receive a total of forty hours of training to know how to appropriately support their future children in the way they need. My husband and I did the entire training and got our home ready for adoption. It was a lot of work and learning. We are not training vulnerable children how to interact with their adoptive parents. The party perceived as more powerful should be trained in supporting the party that actually needs support.

What about a course of study that would include cultural and linguistic acceptance of peers and considerations for the struggles of immigrant peers, such as social isolation, loneliness, cultural differences, and so on. I will repeat: not for the clients—**for our peers at college or at our workplace**. This would be a course directed at peer support so that students know better and will be able to do better. In this case, progress can be about giving people the ability to think about subjects they never thought about before. Formal training like this might have made a difference for Michelle, who became the "go to" girl on all things Latinx at her university, or Pang who took it upon herself to educate her peers and the faculty at her college. I am keeping my fingers crossed that a program chair is reading this book at this moment; these actions don't have to come from our national organization. Every one of you can take this idea right now and start conversations at your workplace or your college—unless you would rather have this book as a required reading assignment at the start of the program for all students.

Heck, I am sure that any minority alumni that finished the graduate program would be happy to give a talk on the subject to new students in any program. I know I would. The point is: information must be given and conversations must be started. Either way, I trust that bringing awareness is one important step, and it must be implemented as early as when everyone is still learning each other's names. Prevention can avoid the need for many of us to write our own books.

The hope here is that eventually these students will become faculty, chair of departments, or any other positions of leadership, and they will be able to arrive at those positions with a better understanding of our struggles as students. Could we go a step further? Sure could. Could we ask ASHA to expand the cultural competency training for faculty to include specific needs of minority and diverse peers? Hello, ASHA friends, this one's for you. You're welcome.

What if we listened to the voices of our minority colleagues when they said what made a difference for them? A few of them, such as Maria Claudia Franca, who had an incredible experience, already gave you guys lots of thoughts on this subject. Here is a word from Jamila:

> **"**I feel I am one of the fortunate clinicians of color in the field. My experience is not common, but it should be. I was fortunate to have a series of divine connections. I had great mentors and peer mentors, and I was connected to influential people in the field. Also, I was connected to NBASLH before I became a student and then during my graduate program. This was an essential component of my success."
> Jamila Perry Harley

If you are faculty, make yourself available and specifically ask minority students to check in with you. For me, that type of support was pivotal. I don't think I could have made it if the faculty that supported me didn't go beyond her role as my educator. I know that I am speaking as a Brazilian student who is more accustomed to building stronger relationships with faculty, but I think your presence and the connection you offer your students is invaluable. Don't wait to be approached by the student. I know I needed that and was too embarrassed to reach out, especially to someone in a position of authority.

In all this, we, the ones who already experienced the effect of bias and microaggression, must be willing to open up to share our experiences. As my therapist would say, "Sometimes it is easier to let things stay in the past and not revisit it. It is easier, but not healthy." I also know that in opening up, we run the risk of being called undiplomatic, ungrateful, or even aggressive. It sucks. However, what if it leads to beautiful connections?

You can use your voice to connect. You can also use your voice to speak up and become an advocate for others. Speaking up and becoming an advocate is not for the faint of heart. We must be able to respect our pain and suffering and be aware that things come in their own time. I have talked about awareness of our trauma being the first step. Some of us will spend years in this phase, and that's okay. You do not have to speak up every chance you get. You do not have to connect with your peers every single time either. Respect your own time. It took me a long time to get to a place where I was finally ready to speak up, challenge expectations, or simply stop being cordial for the sake of cordiality.

If the conversations are with the very people who brought us to a place of pain, things won't be easy. Asking questions or initiating conversations can be triggering, and I've found that many of my friends are not yet at a place where they can dig up those memories. That's okay. Take your time. Keep moving forward. When you feel that you can, go ahead and document, write a blog post, write an email, or ask questions. I emailed both universities I attended asking for information on names for awards. I told them the title of my book, but I have not had any response since. However, I am confident that just by asking questions, people might start paying attention. While I keep my fingers crossed, go ahead and ask your own questions.

More than one person asked me if they could contribute to my book anonymously; one decided to avoid the difficult subject, and the other decided that she was too scared of the repercussions of what she had to share, given the "small SLP world," and decided not to share. The other one, DM, shared, and you read her stories throughout this book. Often, it is not about us not being ready; it is about others not being ready to respect your experience. Assess your truth. You will be ready to speak up one day. Even if you are afraid, like I still am, you may find enough strength to just get it out there.

Online writing was the very first step I took in advocacy as I shared my experiences on my GeekSLP blog. We all have a first step in this journey. We now have a huge platform of colleagues ready to listen, and if you can impact one SLP by sharing your story, that's a win. I hope that you find your own way. In fact, I am sure you will.

Reflection Question: Do you have a person in mind that you can connect with right now?

Chapter 24:

Begin with Grace, but Keep Asking Questions

"Every great dream begins with a dreamer. Always remember, you have within you the strength, the patience, and the passion to reach for the stars to change the world." Harriet Tubman

Writing this book was one of the most taxing emotional experiences I have had (maybe behind graduate school and motherhood). I cried nearly every single day I wrote. I had to ask myself deep questions, digging into areas I had been hiding and pretending didn't bother me anymore. I even questioned the validity of my interpretations of my own experiences. This chapter was completely unplanned; it was born out of two quick-to-judge responses from fellow minority SLPs.

One of the areas that is the hardest is asking if I have shown enough grace to others and the balance between my hurt and someone else's journey. Not everything is about me. As I started the journey of speaking up and opening up about my experiences in this field, especially revisiting things that happened years ago, I understood that I have to tell myself to show some grace. People change and evolve. That's exactly what I wanted to happen to them in the first place. At times, my response to situations has not been the most appropriate. I wish I had shown more grace. I understand that in our trauma responses, we may end up conditioned to assume the worst and quickly make assumptions about the intention of others.

As I have gotten older and a little wiser from all the butt kicking life gave me, I have tried to do better. I have also done better because I have been a victim of quick judgment. People don't ask people to clarify what they mean anymore. The most recent situations happened as I was writing this book. As always, I never waste an opportunity to change the narrative to something useful. Pivot. It inspired me to write this chapter. Thanks! Both stories show a lack of trust among our community, which I introduced in a previous chapter. If we can't trust another minoritized woman, how are we ever going to start healing and building a safe community for everyone?

When I came across the data of male awardees at the 2021 ASHA Convention, I was looking for common ground with ALL women SLPs on the subject. I felt like I had just made an incredible discovery. So, I posted a tweet about how white men were ultimately winning this race within our field. Someone quickly responded to my tweet with accusations of me purposely ignoring the racial aspect and only focusing on the gender issue. That accusation came as I was in the middle of writing a book in which gender is but a chapter. Hello, the bigger purpose of the book is addressing exactly what she accused me of ignoring: racial and ethnic biases.

Advocating is needed. Speaking up is a must. But we must also have the humility to gather all the information before making accusations and assumptions about our colleagues. We must give everyone an opportunity to clarify things. Give people an opportunity to learn that they made a mistake. Give people an opportunity to apologize. Don't get me wrong, I am a person who is big on impact over intention. Sometimes even if people didn't have intention, they still impact us, and we will react. We must be able to trust one another; but at the very least, we must start by asking questions.

What response do you think I had when I was accused in a public forum of racial inappropriateness? I shut down. She didn't ask the question, "Why did you focus on the gender issue?" She directly accused me of racial bias. She assumed things about a random stranger she had never talked to, even online. Sometimes we scream because we are angry and sick and tired of the bullshit. I get it! But that rarely leads to a positive outcome or change in behavior. Isn't that what we ultimately want to see? Yes, we are frustrated, but directing that anger toward someone you know nothing about hurts everyone. It hurts the very cause we want to advance.

Writing this book gave me a glimpse of two sides. Everyone is hurting and mistrusting everyone. This sucks. I do hate the quote, "Hurt people hurt people," because I want us to be a community that helps people. I don't want to believe that we will continue the cycle of hurt. In the process of writing this book, I reached out to anyone in any way I could. I started with my close friends, then expanded to asking them for recommendations. After talking to all of my close friends and their contacts, I realized there were some groups that I still had not spoken to or who still didn't contribute their views on this book: immigrant SLPs, Asian SLPs, and Indigenous SLPs. So I posted a public call to action on my Instagram and also wrote a call to action on Facebook. The final part included reaching out to some specific Instagram accounts. I welcomed anyone and everyone who wanted to contribute.

In one of those interactions on Instagram, I found an account focused on racial and ethnic SLP topics. This account was managed anonymously, and I felt the urge to know more about who was behind it to see if they would be a good fit. In my messages, I said, "Hi, I would love to get to know you. Who runs this account?" to which someone responded, "Good morning, Barbara, what questions can I answer for you?" I immediately felt the wall. Empath alert. So I thought it was a good idea to explain that I was writing a book and came across the account, and since they post a lot on the subject, I wanted to see if they wanted to contribute. Their reply started with, "In scrolling through your content . . ." Then it moved to the fact that one of the admins is "vehemently opposed to being referred to as a minority." Then they commented on the fact that I have two successful businesses and told me that "participating in an interview for a book for profit is providing free labor. We don't see how doing so for someone else's profit is beneficial to us" (referring to speaking to me without a fee). They also told me that if I was interested in their time, we could discuss their consulting fees.

I responded that I understood their position and asked if I should stop asking questions. As you can imagine, the interaction never moved forward. In one reply, what could have been a possible collaboration for constructive growth for an entire industry just ended. Sometimes we are villainized for exclusion. This was the first time I was villainized for inclusion. I welcomed different ideas and opinions, but in return, I was being judged—not for one thing but many aspects, including the fact that I owned two businesses. Was this the fight against capitalism?

This is not related to their request to be paid a fee, but everything else. They expected me to agree to a fee for someone I knew absolutely nothing about. I don't know their gender, race, age, or background. In fact, I knew absolutely nothing about who these people might be. The last message was them saying that I was villainizing their straight response when I said I felt judged. I am not their enemy! We are not each other's enemies! When did we become so quick to push away people who are trying to promote progress?

This book, which started to share my own journey, expanded to be inclusive of others dealing with the same bullshit as I have. My job here is that of a journalist, asking, listening, empathizing, and eventually letting us all be seen.

I was so confused, and honestly, the exchange was mind-boggling. That's when I sent Phuong a text. I needed perspective. That's a humbling exercise. This is what she said:

> "Hi, Barbara. I think there are truths on both ends here. From their perspective, I understand the points they brought up: compensation for their time and the considerations related to profit. I'll be honest, I have responded in a similar fashion when others have asked me to write for them. I think as "minoritized" individuals, there is always a defensiveness because our efforts have been exploited, and this is their boundary setting.
> Which brings me to my next thought . . . Your intention in writing this book is pure. I know this because I know you. To be honest, I only wrote for you because I have a relationship with you. I can understand how this 'ask' can be received if the people do not know you. I hope this brings perspective." Phuong Lien Palafox

Phuong's response is brilliant because she shines a light on things that I assumed as being a mutual understanding between both parties. From my point of view, I am willing to collaborate with people I know to make progress any way we are able to. From their point of view, I was attempting to exploit their time for my own financial profit. The difference is, I wanted to get to know them. Their response was that of someone who thought they knew me—and worse, my intentions. What I am trying to say is: we, as a diverse group, must be able to understand and respect different opinions and ways of thinking. The only way forward is walking through this field without so much pre-judgment. I want to be seen in this field. I want everyone to be seen as well.

Just two months ago, I contributed to a book titled *Becoming an Exceptional SLP*, led by Mai Ling Chan. My contribution was one of fifteen other chapters written by other SLPs. That contribution took hours from my time. None of the contributors were paid for their chapters. I was okay with it. My payment is inspiring other SLPs. Would I have had a problem if all other authors received compensation but I didn't? You bet! All other contributions were voluntary as well. I have been a very well-paid guest speaker. But I have also done it countless times without an honorarium. In my opinion, the issue arises when we are asked to contribute but are treated differently than our white peers—paid less or not paid BECAUSE of our "minority status."

Six months ago, I was approached by a journalist from the *New York Times* about my experience as a person with an accent in our field. I was happy to spend thirty minutes with her on the phone because I want my story to be told. The published story didn't include my piece because of the word count. The journalist eventually told me that her editor had to cut down some stories and mine was one of them. I didn't assume that the journalist was exploiting my time without compensation or excluding me from the article. When the story came out, I saw that there were many more prominent minority people interviewed. I mean, way above my league in many other fields. I give grace. I have given many free presentations, free mentorship, and just last week, I was asked to speak to students in a virtual meeting pro bono; I do it because it is part of my journey.

Does that mean I judge people who always ask for a fee for a chat that might be included in a book? Absolutely not. We are a diverse group. That's exactly how it should be. I want to be accepted in my way of navigating this field as much as I accept anyone else's.

When there is a lack of trust between two minority women, and we start every conversation with deep mistrust among ourselves, how are we going to unite, move forward, and build? I was never asked if the book was for profit or if I was going to donate a portion to the authors—I was asked absolutely nothing. The person/people behind the account can't possibly have an issue with me receiving profits from the book as they are profiting from selling their own paraphernalia promoting diversity. The issue was helping *me* benefit. We are here. Muchachas, find your people who will be open to having conversations without so much judgment.

I want to make something clear: this is not about your personal choice of having a consulting fee. I have my own consulting fee numbers on my website; as my roles have grown, including my role as a mother, I have had to make myself a little less available, so I completely understand. This is about doing to others what we dislike having done to us: quickly judging without much information. If you want to charge, great. If you don't want to charge, that's great too. However, if you want to be the only one among sixteen to get paid while simultaneously refusing to engage when approached, it's hypocritical to claim to be a victim of lack of inclusion.

We need to ask questions, engage, and connect with each other. Shutting down conversations among ourselves is the fastest way to remain even more isolated. In this process the person or people involved in this story pushed me to "validate" their assumptions that (a) I was exploiting their labor by asking if they would like to contribute and (b) that I villainized their request for payment, when on my end, I walked away feeling judged as someone who wanted to exploit them and hurt and villainized for asking my friends for their stories. We all lose.

Do you know who else could have lost? The other people that I might not have invited to participate for fear of a similar reaction (remember my confrontation phobia? LOL). Also, the entire field would have had fewer stories to read about and connect to. Luckily, I had already reached out to many others prior to this incident, and luckily, that was the only confrontational response I received from my many requests.

As I sit here writing, I have already gone through places of fear, wondering about the response I will receive from the 91.5% when my book is out there. I am afraid of the pushback from the people and organizations I spoke about;

I didn't want to have to be afraid of you too. I have had many days while writing this book that I would tell myself, "Barbara, why are you picking up this task? Just let someone else do it." Then I realized that I don't want to be afraid anymore. Nonetheless, it will suck when I start receiving people's "feedback," and I hope they won't tear me down. Especially if the feedback comes after they read the summary version of the book.

In the last chapter of Part Two, I asked for unity and collaboration to help each other shine and thrive. Here, I ask for grace, respect, and going the extra mile to show kindness and respect towards minoritized individuals. I ask you to ask questions before judging each other so abruptly. If this is how we judge the people who are on our own team, and if we question their intentions, how are we going to survive? We need each other!

This has made me think a lot about my past actions, blog posts, tweets, and comments about our professional organizations. We often forget that organizations are composed of human beings. Grouping an entire organization, we might add another barrier to constructive change. Even in this book writing process, I wrote about my issues with ASHA as a whole. I have been considering my approach. ASHA is a giant organization with paid staff and volunteer SLPs. ASHA's staff has several minority SLPs. ASHA volunteers are composed of several minority SLPs. For the last sixteen years, I have seen many of them, some of which I consider my close MSLP alumni friends, go above and beyond to make changes. A lot of the people we talk about have donated their time without any monetary compensation besides the expenses of attending meetings. I have close friends who have dedicated their time, energy, and effort to advocate for a variety of our professional issues and make changes in the organization; these are friends within the minoritized group. When we are angry at a position ASHA as an organization has taken, we often do not direct our voices towards a particular group within ASHA. We generalize. We throw words in the air in hopes that someone catches them. We often don't even take a few minutes to look up details. We just judge. Are we doing the same exact thing that we want people to stop doing to us?

I would like to make a comparison to whatever organization you work within. One of your coworkers could have made a mistake, but because you both work at the same place, you were also blamed for the mistake. This mistake could have been a racial slur or a work-related task. Here I come with my own story, and I am sure you can think of a time when a coworker screwed up big time, and you would not have wanted to be grouped with him or her.

Two years ago, my son was due for his three year reevaluation at his elementary school. Prior to that, they needed my consent to test, right? I called the diagnostician, whom I had worked with a couple times, to tell her that I did not consent to have his IQ tested. My son is a grade skipper and high-performing child; there was no need for an IQ test as this was not an area of concern. I reaffirmed this wish at a meeting I requested prior to refusing to give consent. Then we got busy talking as they printed the document, and I signed while talking, then left. When it was time to have a review meeting, I came to find out that she had tested his IQ. Amiga, I was livid! I wrote to the principal, special education director, and even the superintendent. However, I can't imagine making a positive impact if I wrote blaming the entire district for that gross and absurd error by the diagnostician. I wanted them to hold her accountable. If you as the SLP were also blamed for her mistake, I am sure that would have been a hard pill to swallow. What I am trying to say here is . . . in the age of advocacy, in which we can write blog posts or blast entire organizations for a mistake, we must also make an effort to be as just and fair as we can. We want to promote change. I am not contradicting myself and telling you to be diplomatic. You better believe when I tell you that I was far from diplomatic. However, I made sure to direct my anger towards the right people and make sure that whoever could hold the person accountable also saw how furious I would be if actions were not taken. My son's school does a lot of wonderful things for him. I was not going to throw away the baby with the bath water.

I will save your disagreement and be my own devil's advocate; as a business owner, I will take the responsibility for one of my employee's mistakes. I do not expect you to direct your anger towards my developer when the app crashes. This works because I am the owner of two tiny businesses. I doubt that the staff who work for ASHA in multicultural issues is made aware of what ASHA's healthcare conference is putting together and vice versa; at least not in detail. Maybe they should talk. But are SLPs who work at a preschool aware of what fifth-grade teachers do? Not really. Being crumpled together when someone makes a mistake will only hurt the laser target actions needed for change.

When I started my business, my illustrator was based in the Philippines. I love her work. It is cute and creative. She created illustrations for an articulation app called *Articulate Plus*. After a while, I started to notice that she had a variety of illustrations with people with purple, green, or pink hair; but I could not find one person who had darker skin or who was Black. I was able to correct the discrepancy in representation as we continued the illustration process, but in that, I had an aha moment. The Black population in the Philippines accounts for less than 0.01% of the population. That's one tenth of a percent. I didn't immediately jump the gun on her. I understood that I had to specifically make requests about what I wanted to see, without judgment. We were able to continue the work, and since then, she has made sure to make Smarty Ears illustrations diverse.

Earlier this week, I saw a post about the lack of diversity on a product from a large publisher in our field. Obviously, that company has hundreds of employees, while I have only a handful. There were times in which it was not an option for me to actually have options of diversity in my images. I am sure that even though I never received an email, I could have been judged for not having much diversity. When I released my first app twelve years ago, I didn't have a budget to hire my own illustrator. I was licensing images from an affordable image bank. I was very aware of the lack of diversity; any time I had a photo of a human, the person was Caucasian. Except for rare exceptions, I was never able to find diversity in that image bank. As my business grew, I was able to afford licensing images from a more premium image bank or hire my own illustrator for my apps. As a small business owner, I was feeling the trickle-down effect of a larger business's lack of diversity awareness. It has looked great to sound "woke" and criticize companies, but unless you knew me and knew the whole story, you might have judged me and my business too. Obviously, we live in different times, where it is much easier to tackle this issue, but I could have been crucified in the beginning of my business if social media looked anything like it does today.

In continuation of being my own devil's advocate: would anyone have noticed the lack of different shades of skin on those adorable illustrations if Smarty Ears was not owned by a minority SLP? These days, probably—

twelve years ago, I am not sure. I believe in the magic that can be created when we are able to look at the same thing and see it in a completely different light.

I am calling on you to go beyond quick judgment and quick, "woke" social media posts and take a few minutes to ask questions or be open to listen to other people's perspectives without putting up a wall. We need each other!

We already have enough people tearing us down. We can build ourselves up. Remember what happened in 2016? Women marched in protest. But do you also remember what happened in 2018? Women ran for office in record numbers. We can protest and write our opinions online, but I am calling on you to drive change. You don't have to run for office; you can do it your way.

Chapter 25:

Driving Progress Your Way

"I learned a long time ago the wisest thing I can do is be on my own side, be an advocate for myself and others like me.**"**
Maya Angelou

I used to feel guilty every time I got a chance to hang and hear updates about some of my MSLP girls. Many of them are serving in real positions of leadership. Amiga, many of these positions are volunteer positions! These women have full-time jobs and have found the time and energy to engage and contribute. For the many reasons I explained previously, including my personality style and my absolute aversion to bureaucracy, chain of command, and procedures, I could never contribute or take an active role within associations, which is how we drive policy changes. There are many of you out there with talent for this type of impact. These days, as an expert on my own strengths and weaknesses, I know that I have contributed to the promotion of diversity in this field in my own style. I did it my way, and I want you to do it your way, so in this chapter, I want to share with you a few ways in which I have made these contributions.

Just earlier this week, I jumped on a meeting with Dr. Kia Johnson, current chair of NBASLH, about an idea I had to increase the number of minority women in innovation and businesses in our field. In order to implement my vision, we would need to recruit another more organized SLP to execute all that needed to be done in terms of organization and preparation. I am not that person. While this is an important issue for me, enough for me to volunteer hours of my time, I am fully aware of my limitations when it comes to planning. As a highly impatient person, projects that are "not now," that need the approval of multiple individuals, are absolutely beyond my capacity. I understand that we each should contribute in building each other in the way we can and are able to. I have found my way to contribute, and I want you to find yours. Your unique perspective and talents will bring light to areas of need in this field in ways that others can't.

Several years ago, when I had the idea to implement the character of choice feature within my symbol set, Smarty Symbols, I was initially driven by the awareness of the fact that all existing symbol set characters were white male stick figures, and there were no female representations. So, my first character was Violet. Creating thousands of symbols is no small task. It took my two illustrators months to fully create all images of Violet (a girl with light skin tone). As we were in the process of creating those images, I decided to create more characters with other skin shades. As I had that idea, I decided to reach out to the one person within my network who worked her entire life as an AAC advocate to ask her thoughts on creating different representations for my symbol set. She responded that she didn't see a need for that because the stick figures of the existing symbol sets were not white; they were "colorless." She is a progressive, older Caucasian woman. Her response and perception of those stick figures surprised me. I have a lot of respect for her, and considered her an AAC queen. I ignored her suggestion nonetheless. I went ahead and created my new diverse symbol.

Smarty Symbols has several diverse characters that allow clinicians and educators to create an entire communication board or AAC device pages with a character that more closely represents each student. I am proud to say that I believe my innovation in symbol set diversity contributed a lot to how other symbol sets have recently implemented the ability to change skin tone on their stick figure. I believe we are more than our skin tone, which is why I created entire new characters for Smarty Symbols. This process took years worth of work, and for a small business, this was a major undertaking. My symbol set is still a work in progress as I plan to continue to drive innovation.

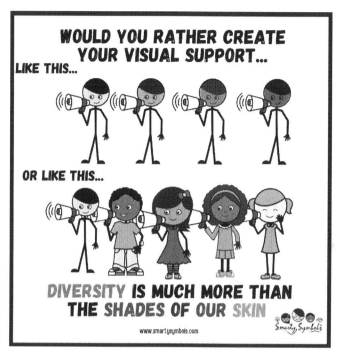

Instagram post from @smartysymbols

I absolutely believe that it was my initiative to create a diverse symbol with my "character of choice" option that drove an entire industry towards a more inclusive and diverse offering by my competitors. Even the fact that I had a female character as a default was innovative. Sexism in visual representation? That's for you to decide.

Despite the fact that I have contributed so much via technology, I believe that introducing diversity in visual support will be my biggest contribution to the world. Nonetheless, I doubt that I will ever be recognized for this contribution. The AAC industry has not had their status quo challenged much; and making space for new innovative contributions from "outsiders" has rarely been seen.

If you are a more organized, planner type, run for office. ASHA has several positions available, so you can contribute in many different roles. Did you get upset that your presentation proposal was not accepted? Ask how you can become a reviewer the following year. You can volunteer for both

ASHA and your own state convention. I have served two times as a reviewer for ASHA's convention proposals in two areas. This year, I was invited again to review proposals for the telepractice group. I can say that this is an area I am definitely not cut out for. Reading proposals and determining the potential for a presentation was hard work, and it was an unpaid volunteer position. In fact, I was a reviewer for one of the NIH grant rounds, and I knew I could never do that again. That's just not one of my strengths. I have also served as a member of the Texas Speech and Hearing Association Cultural and Linguistic Diversity Task Force for two years—another unpaid volunteer contribution. ASHA has a variety of volunteer positions available. Now, you can also apply for one of the paid positions. There is currently an opening for Chief Staff Officer for Multicultural Affairs, and the salary is wow! By the time this book gets to your eyes, this position might have been filled. But if you are looking to make a change from within, go ahead and look at ASHA's career page.

Mentorship is another area that I could have been highlighting throughout this book. There are several official programs such as the STEP program that you can volunteer for. This goes both ways—if you need a mentor or if you want to be a mentor. Mentorship does not have to be official. It can be a sincere, supportive chat at a convention, a text message, or a call to someone you can help. It is that simple. We need each other!

If you are good with technology, you can contribute by creating online courses to increase awareness and promote change. Many of us have created online communities geared towards minority SLPs. Just this week, a group of SLPs led by Ebony Green held a virtual conference called, "Black SLPs in Private Practice." Create a course geared toward cultural sensitivity, toward culturally diverse SLPs or SLP students, or courses to empower diverse SLPs. You can also write your own book, share your story in a blog post, write an article, or submit your writing to publications.

If you are a business owner, consider sponsoring activities that support multicultural themes. Smarty Ears has been a sponsor of many multicultural events over the last ten years, including the NBASLH convention. I will confess that my lack of organization is the reason I have not done more; luckily, people have reached out to me. You can also donate to the MSLP program, which was pivotal for many of us in finding belonging.

As a businesswoman and owner of a small business, I have found that it was important to me to make my apps available in several languages but especially in Portuguese. I rarely make back the investment because there are not enough Brazilian speakers in the US receiving therapy in Portuguese. In Brazil, the iPad was adopted in therapy at much lower rates in comparison to the US. However, linguistic accessibility to my creation is part of my legacy in this field. Smarty Symbols is available in eight languages, and users can create visual support resources in any of those eight languages with the touch of a button without even knowing the language. I have given presentations at Brazilian universities free of charge because I want to empower them to make a difference. I want them to see their worth. I want them to know how our education in Brazil is incredibly comprehensive, especially compared with the US training. I am extremely vigilant about the art my team creates for my apps to make sure it includes and represents minorities. I created the first bilingual assessment of articulation and phonology that actually tests both languages in one product, both in Portuguese (AFAP) and Spanish (BAPA).

I also contribute as a Brazilian SLP in my community. I have spent hours on the phone supporting Brazilian parents as they navigate the special education system, finding services, initiating assessments, explaining assessment results, and guiding them on supporting their child. Many of the Brazilians in my community don't speak English yet, as recent immigrants, or didn't attend school here, so I help them navigate that process. My name is known in the Dallas - Ft. Worth Brazilian community as the "Fonoaudiologa" who does not practice or provide therapy anymore but can support. So they reach out, and I am available on the phone as much as possible. I do not receive any compensation. I do this because I care, and I want to support them as much as I wish I had support for myself.

I have done and contributed a lot. I have contributed in ways I haven't even shared in this book. I have contributed to this field my way. I want you to find your way too. I know you will.

Reflection Question: What traits of your personality would be most important in finding a way to contribute to driving progress?

Barbara Fernandes

Chapter 26:

Closing Thoughts

"If you suffered in life and want other people to suffer as you did because 'you turned out fine,' you did not in fact turn out fine."
Daniel Swensen

This book changed me, and I'm glad it did. Reflecting is a big part of growing. It is what makes awareness possible, and awareness is our first step to healing. Regardless of whether or not you find the energy, time, calling, or strength to make change, there is one thing I beg you to start doing that is even more important than contributing: healing. In healing, you will find acceptance of the whole you. I am not there yet; I still can't stand the sound of my own voice on the videos I made, and I never rewatch them specifically because of that. That's the journey I am on. Nonetheless, you may hear it for hours if I decide to record an audio version of this book. Healing takes time. We heal a little with each action. My self-awareness grows with each vulnerable engagement, so I choose to be vulnerable whenever possible.

As I wrote this book, I became aware that, as much as I tried once, I can't run away from many parts of my culture and language. I could never afford books in Brazil. I started attempting to read in Portuguese much later in life, as I could actually afford books when I got my job as an SLP. Books from Brazilian authors have these page-long paragraphs that drove me absolutely insane. From my observations, book reading is still not something that is part of the Brazilian mainstream culture for leisure. It is still a very elitist activity; so the writing is always very complex and snobbish, in my opinion, with rare exceptions, unless you are reading true classics. Despite all this, and despite being very conscious about my language tendencies, I still wrote long paragraphs as I wrote this book; especially when I was writing emotional stories. I say all that to say, even the parts of my culture that I don't like are ingrained in my behavior. That awareness and acceptance is freeing, nonetheless. You can thank the editors that you didn't have to try to figure out my long sentences. I choose to be aware of the influence of my language and culture.

I will never know if I would have found the inspiration to become an author if it weren't for the negative experiences I still face that push me to speak up louder. The lesson that I learned from one person could have ended with me, but it didn't. My voice now resonates with a much bigger number of people than just myself. How is that for a good diplomatic answer? As my colleague Dr. Teresa Girolamo told me, "I turned shit into fertilizer." I have grown from this book, and I hope you grew with me. I choose to grow and learn from my experiences.

There were many moments when I almost didn't make it. There were moments in which I almost gave up. I almost sold my businesses a few times. I have even approached my husband on many occasions in tears saying, "I can't do this anymore. Let's just sell it all and move overseas!" I don't believe in destiny, but as Paulo Coelho (1993) would say:

> **"** . . . and when you really want something, all the universe always conspires in helping you achieve it." *The Alchemist*

So much of what happened in my life felt like the universe was conspiring in my favor. All the people who touched my life seemed to appear when I most needed them. All the people who came back for me when they arrived to where they were going often had no idea of their impact on me or all the amazing things I would achieve one day. Even the doors that closed were simply showing me the way to living a life that speaks to my soul every single day. Good or bad, it didn't matter! The sale that fell through, the bad business decisions, the negative interactions . . . all of that led me here just so I could be here for you too. I choose to show up for others whenever possible.

"When you finally arrive where you were going. Look back and help her too. Because there was a time that you were her." Unknown author (n.d.)

It is often said that diamonds are made under pressure. We have had more than our fair share of pressure in this field that might have propelled us into the diamonds we are today. However, I am not sure if the pressure I endured was worth it, even when entertaining the idea that it was this pressure that turned me into the kick-ass woman I am today. I am not sure if I would have picked to experience the suffering and trauma I did, even if that's the reason I achieved so much in this field. One could argue that the psychology of "having something to prove to them" pushed me further and further up, and that I may not have achieved half as much without so much pressure and struggle. I honestly don't know, amiga.

However, here is something that I know: when I think about my daughter, who has more melanin in her skin than me, I do *not* want to see her soul crushed as mine was. She is strong and amazing exactly as she is and does not need someone else's pressure or standards to make her into a better version of herself. I do not wish this for my daughter, so likely, I would not wish that on myself either.

I've achieved a lot. Sometimes I even look back and say, "Wow." It took a lot to do it. I can still feel every second of the long grueling hours studying, working, dreaming, and building that it took to get here. That said, my effort wasn't everything. People helped me get where I am today. I am grateful for the ones who came before me and helped make the steps of change. Don't kick down the ladder you came up on. If anything, help build more ladders.

I do not want to take away my own credit for reaching and breaking all the glass ceilings I did, or minimize the efforts of my father or all the other people that have contributed in small or large ways to my journey. However, one of the biggest contributors to the fact that I am living the wonderful life I get to experience today is the fact that I was born into a society that allowed me to pursue a higher education at a government-funded institution. Brazil, as a developing country, has a lot of growth to do, especially regarding income inequality and social mobility, but we have high-quality free public higher education. Through governmental initiatives, my country also sponsored the first six months of my stay abroad, and it was through that experience that my worldview completely changed. They invested in me so I could keep all of us moving forward. I learned through personal experience to allow myself to accept that different people have different values. It was through the process of stepping away from my country that I could see how much of my culture I will always carry with me.

I will forever carry gratitude for the women who have paved the way for me, like the women who started an SLP program at my college in Brazil—I was in the third graduating SLP class—or the women who created the exchange student program to bring me to the USA. I also have to mention the Brazilian women who wanted to support other Brazilians, the women who created and organized each year of the MSLP program, and the women who supported me as I navigated life. These women had no idea that one day, I would cross their lives, and I would go on to make my own impact in our field. I honor them and will always remember them. These wonderful women are what came to my mind when I heard Kamala Harris's VP acceptance speech: "While I may be the first woman in this office," Harris vowed, "I will not be the last because every little girl watching tonight sees that this is a country of possibilities." For me, I felt a weight and responsibility that Kamala must feel to make sure she wasn't the last. Only others who have thought to themselves, "How do we pave this path so that others won't struggle so much for this stretch of the journey?" can really understand a moment like this. I think she understands this weight and responsibility to do her best to make sure the torch continues beyond herself and ensure that progress does not end. I feel this weight, as well. I know "the firsts" who came before me helped me be a first in a different way. The "firsts" that I can accomplish make a pathway for those who will come after me and make their own "firsts." We know that many important people, with important gifts to offer humanity, are still coming. Let's make sure they can get here safely.

I didn't cover everything. How could I? I'm just one person. I tried my best to include friends that also had important stories and perspectives to share. I even made myself vulnerable and tried to reach beyond the comfort of my own circle to include even more diversity and the important perspectives that come with it. In the end, I know there is more to tell—a lot more—and I hope you continue the journey of telling it. More truths need to be spoken. Movements are never fully truthful when they focus on the one "hero" leader instead of the movement of the people who came together to make it an unstoppable wave of change—each contributing in their own way.

Now amiga, go make progress!

Barbara

Barbara Fernandes

About the Voices in This Book

Barbara Fernandes, MS, CCC-SLP

Barbara Fernandes, an award-winning Brazilian American speech-language pathologist, immigrated to the United States as an adult with very limited English skills. She went on to become one of the most successful entrepreneurs in her field, founding two businesses and revolutionizing her field with nearly seventy successful product launches to date.

As the founder and CEO of Smarty Ears, she is well known for her innovative and breakthrough product development for speech and communication disorders. For over a decade, Barbara has translated science into user friendly and powerful technology to support individuals with communication disorders. Barbara transformed an entire industry to adopt mobile technologies through the design and development of over sixty mobile applications and an entire symbol library: Smarty Symbols.

As the founder of Smarty Symbols, Barbara also created the most inclusive, diverse, and comprehensive symbol library and developed a powerful new technology that is disrupting the special education field by providing a platform for custom visual support creation. Smarty Symbols has been adopted as the symbol of choice in many other technologies developed in the field.

Through her blog and video podcast, Barbara became known as GeekSLP. Barbara has traveled the country to train special education professionals in the adoption of mobile technology to promote student learning and engagement. She has been a guest speaker in multiple state association conventions, the national American Speech-Language and Hearing convention, as well as the Brazilian and Canadian conventions.

Most recently, Barbara has been awarded a Small Business Innovation Research (SBIR) grant by the National Institute of Health, and she released a ground-breaking technology called the Speech and Language Academy. Barbara has received multiple awards, and is an Amazon best-selling author.

Contact:

Instagram: @GeekBarbara
Twitter: @GeekBarbaraSLP
TikTok: @geekbarbara
Email: bfernandes@smartyearsapps.com
Linkedin: https://www.linkedin.com/in/bfernanddes/

Websites:

Personal: www.barbarafernandes.com
Smarty Ears: www.smartyearsapps.com
Speech Language Academy: www.speechlanguageacademy.com
Smarty Symbols: www.smartysymbols.com

QR code with direct contact links:

D.M., MS, CCC-SLP (Anonymous contributor)
Contributor, D.M., is a close friend who was afraid of the retaliation she might experience for speaking truth to power and has decided to contribute anonymously. I will honor her words and vulnerability and hope that people like her won't have to hide their truth again.

Ebony Green, MS, CCC-SLP
Ebony Green is an African-American/Belizean-American bilingual speech language pathologist in the Phoenix area. Ebony is a former member of Teach for America with a background in elementary and secondary education. Ebony is a first generation college graduate and the daughter of an immigrant mother and American father. Ebony owns a private practice in

Arizona, and she is the Founder of The SLP Business Suite, an online learning community for speech language pathologists interested in entrepreneurship and leadership development.

Enjoli M. Richardson, MS, CCC-SLP

Enjoli M. Richardson is a first-generation college student from Port Arthur, Texas and certified speech-language pathologist. She received her bachelor's degree in Communication Studies from Texas State University-San Marcos and a master's degree in Speech-Language Pathology from Lamar University. Currently, Enjoli is a PhD student with clinical and research interests in exploring stuttering within culturally and linguistically diverse populations. Amongst her affiliations and service within the profession, she is a member of the National Black Association for Speech-Language and Hearing (NBASLH). She is passionate about the next generation of advocacy, mentorship, and cultural responsiveness within CSD, improving support for students of color, and the implementation of antiracist pedagogy.

Jamila Perry Harley, EdM, CCC-SLP

Jamila has a BA in Communication from the University of NC at Chapel Hill and a M.Ed. (Magna Cum Laude) in Communication Sciences and Disorders from North Carolina Central University. Currently, she is a staff member at ASHA, serving as Associate Director for Health Care Services in Speech-Language Pathology. Additionally, she is still actively involved in volunteerism in the profession, including serving as NBASLH's Co-Editor of the Resound Publication and as a member of the Council of Academic Programs in Communication Sciences and Disorders (CAPCSD) Diversity, Equity, and Inclusion Committee. She is passionate about supporting students of color in CSD, DEI in the field of CSD, and leadership development for clinicians of color.

Leila Regio, BA

Leila Regio (she/they/siya) is of Pilipinx (Austronesian/South East Asian), Punjabi-Indian (South Asian), and Chinese (East Asian) descent with high proficiency in their native language, Tagalog (Pilipinx mainstream), basic proficiency in Ilokano and Pangasinense (Pilipinx languages), and basic proficiency in Mandarin (Chinese). Siya identifies as non-binary/queer. Siya graduated with a bachelor's in CSD at California State University, Los

Angeles where siya continues to pursue their master's in Speech-Language Pathology, '22. Leila was invited to speak for the ASHA 2021 Convention's master class on gender affirming voice care alongside fellow trans and gender non-confirming (TGNC) colleagues as co-panelists. Siya is a 2019 alumni of the ASHA Minority Student Leadership Program (MSLP) currently serving as National NSSLHA's Vice President for Student State Officers (Western Region including Hawaii and Puerto Rico), ASHA's Committee of Ambassadors (CoA). Leila seeks to empower students and professionals to commit to culturally responsive care in and out of the clinical setting, engage in grassroots advocacy, and find and support diverse communities, and share resources.

Mai Ling Chan, MS, CCC-SLP
Mai Ling is an American-born Colombian/Chinese speech-language pathologist, industry historian, global connector, and technology entrepreneur. Building on sixteen years of clinical experience, she focuses on supporting disability-focused thought leaders and creating digital products that make a difference in the global special education ecosystem. She is actively involved in several local communities, including women in business, Asian Corporate Entrepreneurial Leaders, assistive technology groups, and is the founder of an Arizona-based speech pathologist Facebook group, which has grown to 1K members.

Contact: www.mailingchan.com

Maria Claudia Franca, PhD, CCC-SLP
Maria Claudia Franca is an endowed professor in the Communication Disorders and Sciences Program at Southern Illinois University with areas of interest in multicultural and global issues related to communication disorders, voice science, and higher education. She has continuously been the instructor of record in dynamic courses designed to increase multicultural awareness and skills among future professionals. Participation in the Minority Student Leadership Program (MSLP) was a turning point for her leadership-focused educational experience. Franca is also an ASHA Diversity Champion. Maria Claudia has been recipient of the Diversity Excellence Award and the Provost Faculty Fellowship at Southern Illinois University for her extensive work in multicultural matters, including regarding first generation college

students. Her achievements have been supported by the University Women's Professional Advancement and Women's Studies at the university. She collaborates at national/international levels and regularly holds leadership appointments at the ASHA and the Illinois Speech-Language-Hearing Association, where she is the current president-elect.

Michelle Hernandez, MS, CCC-SLP

Michelle Hernandez is a first-generation college student and immigrant from the Dominican Republic and certified speech-language pathologist. She has a bachelor's in Psychology and Women's Studies from Stony Brook University and a master's degree in Speech-Language Pathology from SUNY Buffalo State. Michelle is a Bronx native but currently lives in Houston, TX. She is a PhD student with clinical and research interests in bilingual development, bilingual children with language disorders, and code-switching within Spanish-English school-aged children. She also continues to practice in the home health setting and supervises SLPAs. Michelle is committed to translating research to practice to promote effective identification, access, and inclusion for bilingual children who experience communication difficulties.

Michelle Posner, MS, CCC-SLP

Michelle Posner is a bilingual speech-language pathologist in the Washington DC Metropolitan area. She was born in Mexico City and moved to the US when she was nine years old. The combination of these experiences propelled Michelle to pursue a degree in speech-language pathology and to change the narrative. Her experience ranges from private practice and outpatient hospital to school-based SLP in Texas, Florida, Virginia, and DC. Michelle is the founder of BilingualSLP LLC, a company dedicated to providing wrap-around services for bilingual professionals and families. BilingualSLP LLC supports other bilingual SLPs with quality therapy materials, provides consultation services for families raising bilingual children, speaks at daycares on the topic of bilingualism, and much more. This is Michelle's way of making a change for the better.

Website: BilingualSLP.com

Pelesia A. Fields, MS, CCC-SLP

Pelesia A. Fields is a bilingual speech-language pathologist currently based in Loganville, Georgia where she owns a private pediatric speech clinic. Pelesia is a Kenyan native who migrated to the United States as a teenager. She received both her bachelor's and master's degrees in speech-language pathology from Lehman College of the City University of New York. Pelesia holds the Certificate of Clinical Competence through the American Speech-Language-Hearing Association. She is also licensed by the Georgia State Board of Examiners as well as the state of New York. Pelesia holds a post master's advanced graduate certificate in educational leadership from Stony Brook University (New York). Pelesia's professional experiences have given her vast knowledge of language development and use across the communication continuum as well as her understanding of diversity, varied cultures, and language differences.

Ramya Kumar, MS, CCC-SLP (BCS-S, CNT, IBCLC)
Ramya Kumar is of Indian descent and grew up in the United Arab Emirates. She came to the US for her undergraduate degree in Psychology from the University of Massachusetts Lowell. Ramya stayed on at UMASS Lowell for a Masters in Biological Sciences. After a career in higher education she went back to school and graduated from Baylor University with her second masters in Communication Sciences and Disorders. She is currently a neonatal therapist specializing in feeding and swallowing disorders. As a certified Trauma Informed Professional, Ramya is passionate about viewing family dynamics and patient care from the lens of trauma stewardship and cultural competence. She truly believes that each individual—however big or small—brings their story to the mealtime. It is our duty and responsibility as communication specialists to put these stories together, with the aim of creating mealtime success and family centered care.

Website: www.ramyakumarslp.com

Tamala Close, MS, CCC-SLP
Tamala H. Close is a Dallas, Texas native who received her undergraduate degree in CSD from the University of Houston and a graduate degree from the illustrious Southern University A & M's Speech-Language Pathology Program. She is also the founder of SLP Private Practice in Color, a community-based platform for speech-language pathologists from varying cultural backgrounds to exchange resources, network, and mentor clinicians

who made the decision to pursue entrepreneurship and form their own private practice. Currently, SLP Private Practice in Color has expanded to provide professional development that focuses on providing efficacious intervention to individuals from culturally and linguistically diverse backgrounds.

Pang Tao Moua, MS, CF-SLP
Pang Tao Moua is a first-generation Hmong American PhD student in the Department of Communication Sciences and Disorders at the University of Utah. Pang received her bachelor's degree at the University of Wisconsin-River Falls and her Master's degree at the University of Utah in Communication Sciences and Disorders. Pang's research interest focuses on bilingual language assessment of Asian tonal-speaking populations, particularly Hmong. In addition, she also works at a Title 1 school as a speech-language pathologist. Pang is dedicated to increasing support for students of color in CSD, advocating for culturally and linguistically diverse communities seeking speech and language therapy, and promoting cultural responsiveness in the practice of speech-language pathology.

Phuong Lien Palafox, MS, CCC-SLP
Phuong Lien Palafox is a Vietnamese-Chinese bilingual speech-language pathologist, author, and advocate. Currently, her time is spent serving clients and their families, SLPs, and educators across the United States. With a foundation of evidence-based and human-centered practices, she is continually invested in Cultural Responsiveness, Advocacy, Narrative-Based Interventions, and the Mental Health of Educators. She is the author of *The Heartbeat of Speech-Language Pathology*. Attendees leave her presentations and storytellings feeling validated, refueled, and re-engaged to fuel their meaningful work.

Yarimar I. Díaz Rodríguez, MS, CCC-SLP
Yarimar I. Díaz Rodríguez is a doctoral student in the Applied Cognitive Neuroscience Program at Universidad Maimónides in Buenos Aires, Argentina. She is a Certified Bilingual Speech Language Pathologist, born and raised in Puerto Rico. She is licensed in the United States with the state of Florida and US territory Puerto Rico and experienced in evaluation, treatment and investigating methods to improve clinical management of neurological disorders, symptomatic behaviors, including expertise in

Traumatic Brain Injury (TBI) in pediatric and geriatric population. Emerging from Puerto Rico, her greatest challenge is in helping to improve the livelihoods of developing innovative healthcare organizations and industries through sustainable development and innovative leadership principles. Her professional career goal is to promote, as a researcher individual, the use of informatic data and development of the community needs, collaboration, and relationship to the Hispanic community in the United States of America.

Email: yarimar.diaz@outlook.com

Yao Du, PhD, CCC-SLP
Yao Du is a bilingual Mandarin-English speaking speech-language pathologist, a human-computer interaction researcher, and an amateur game designer. She currently works as an assistant professor and clinical supervisor in Speech-Language Pathology at Monmouth University in New Jersey, where she conducts research in areas of telehealth, bilingual assessment, and voice assistants such as Amazon Alexa. She has clinical experiences working in private practices, private schools, skilled nursing facilities, hospitals, and home health and also holds the Advanced Telehealth Coordinator Certificate from the University of Delaware. Additionally, she enjoys offering accent coaching services to Mandarin-English speakers, training special educators and clinical practitioners internationally, and providing consultations to startup companies in digital therapeutics and assistive technology.

Contact: https://www.linkedin.com/in/yaod

References

Aberjhani. (n.d.). *Splendid Literarium: A Treasury of Stories, Aphorisms, Poems, and Essays.*

Andersen, H. C. (1843). *The Ugly Duckling.* Denmark : C.A. Reitzel.

Angelou, M. (1969). *I Know Why the Caged Bird Sings.* Random House Publishing Group.

ASHA. (2021). *2021 ASHA Awards Recipients.* Retrieved from ASHA: https://www.asha.org/about/awards/2021-awards-recipients/

Bossidy, L., & Charan, R. (2002). *Execution: The Discipline of Getting Things Done.* Crown Business.

Britannica, T. Editors of Encyclopedia (2019, September 18). minority. Encyclopedia Britannica. https://www.britannica.com/topic/minority

Bureau, U. S. (2018, December 6). *American Community Survey 2013-2017 5-year Data Release.* Retrieved from United States Census Bureau: https://www.census.gov/newsroom/press-kits/2018/acs-5year.html

Chopra, D. (n.d.).

Christopher, L. 2015, October 1. *Vulnerability is the essence of connection and connection is the essence of existence.* Twitter. https://twitter.com/leo_words/status/649453990854426624

Coelho, P. (1993). *The Alchemist.* HarperTorch.

Hallowell, E.M., & Ratey, J.J. (2021). *ADHD 2.0: New Science and Essential Strategies for Thriving with Distraction--from Childhood through Adulthood.* Ballantine Books.

Harris, K. 2020, November 8. *While I may be the first woman in this office, I will not.* Twitter. https://twitter.com/kamalaharris/status/1325251050509639681

J-1 visa. (2021, November 6). Retrieved from Wikipedia: https://en.wikipedia.org/wiki/J-1_visa

Jemison, M. (n.d.).

Kapin, A. (2019, January 28). *10 Stats That Build The Case For Investing In Women-Led Startups*. Retrieved from Forbes: https://www.forbes.com/sites/allysonkapin/2019/01/28/10-stats-that-build-the-case-for-investing-in-women-led-startups/?sh=d4a934c59d5f

Knowles, B. (2014, January 14). *Beyonce: Gender equality is a myth*. Retrieved from CNN: https://edition.cnn.com/2014/01/13/showbiz/celebrity-news-gossip/beyonce-feminism-shriver-report/index.html

Labor Force Statistics from the Current Population Survey. (2021, January 22). Retrieved from U.S. Bureau of labor statistics: https://www.bls.gov/cps/cpsaat11.htm

Miles, A.L. (2015). *Recovering is an Art*. CreateSpace Independent Publishing Platform.

Miller, H. (1939). *Tropic of Capricorn*. Paris: Obelisk Press.

Niemöller, M. (2020, May). First They Came for the Socialists. *Academic Medicine:*, 95(5), 738. doi: 10.1097/ACM.0000000000003009

Plantinga, C.N. (n.d.).

Rivera, G. (2016). *Juliet Takes a Breath: The Graphic Novel*. BOOM! Box.

Tzu, L. (1868). Tao Te Ching.

60817114R00130